Praise for *The hCG Diet Quick Start Cookbook*

"As an experienced practitioner of the hCG treatment protocol, I highly recommend Anne Wolfinger's book. Her research and insights into this program will benefit anyone in their efforts to find a successful outcome to the hCG diet."

Dr. Michael Bergkamp, ND

The hCG Diet Quick Start Cookbook

30 Days to a Thinner You

Anne Wolfinger

www.hcgdietquickstart.com

AWA Publishing

First Printing, 2012

ISBN 1475252005

Printed in the United States of America

Acknowledgement

Many thanks to Chef Liz Scott for her professional expertise and creativity.

Contents

Chapter Nine

Appendix 1

Introduction

After three friends told me about their hCG diet success, I decided it was time for me to look into it. The first friend was Bonnie. She had lost a very noticeable 40 pounds over two courses of hCG and was planning to do a third. It was impressive. I happened to mention her to Stevie when she next cut my hair. "I lost 20 pounds on hCG," she reported. "I'm on my feet all day too and did just fine with the diet."

But Emma was the one who really got me thinking. She used it to lose 25 pounds before her son's wedding. "I was skeptical at first," Emma told me, "but I researched it pretty well online and decided to give it a try." Emma is a registered nurse, so I figured if it was good enough for her it was a legitimate option.

With the help of a naturopathic physician, I lost 17 pounds my first round in the fall of 2011, gained some back over Christmas, then dropped another 12 in my second round. What amazed me the most was how quickly it happened, and where the weight came off.

I've never been fat, but I'm short (5'4"), pear-shaped, and muscular. My mother tells me I was a "sturdy" child. I'm athletic and active, but I also have a desk job and sometimes don't get the amount of exercise I need each week to eat the way I like to. The scale was slowly but relentlessly trending upward. I was not happy about it, but starting to feel resigned to middle age spread.

Cancel that. I've lost weight in my abdomen, hips and thighs, even my upper arms. hCG has produced results that months of weight-lifting routines and aerobic workouts couldn't touch. Believe me, I've tried.

I'm happy, slender, and determined to stay that way.

That's my success story.

What will be yours?

Chapter One: The Skinny on hCG

What is hCG?

The acronym "hCG" stands for the human chorionic gonadotrophin hormone, and yes, it is properly spelled *hCG*.

The hCG diet was developed in the 1950s by British endocrinologist Dr. Albert T. W. Simeons. Dr Simeons theorized that (1) obesity is a disorder, (2) that abnormal fat is always caused by obesity, (3) that obesity is not caused by overeating but overeating is caused by obesity, (4) that if you suffer from obesity you will get fat no matter how much you eat, and (5) the opposite for those obnoxious and lucky folks we all know, that no matter how much they eat, they don't become overweight because they don't have the obesity disorder.

Dr. Simeons identified three different kinds of fat. Structural fat protects the body's joints and organs. Normal fat is spread all over the body and serves as normal reserves of fuel for activity and maintenance of body temperature. Abnormal fat is the body's last line of defense against starvation. It is stored in your waist, hips, thighs, abdomen, and upper arms—those areas that are annoyingly resistant to change despite typical dieting and targeted exercises. Now you know why.

Dr. Simeons was certain that the problem resided in the hypothalamus gland in the brain. The next trick was to find out how to solve the problem.

His breakthrough came after studying and observing thin pregnant women in India on calorie deficient diets who nevertheless delivered healthy, normal weight babies. Through research, he determined this was the effect of hCG which is naturally produced by the body during pregnancy and affects the hypothalamus gland in the brain, forcing the body to utilize the nutrients stored in the abnormal body fat.

After years of ongoing research and experimentation working with thousands of patients, he developed his weight loss technique, which combined daily doses of hCG with a strict, very low calorie diet.

The hCG Diet

There are three phases to the hCG diet. Phase I is the Loading Phase and lasts the first two days you start taking hCG. In the Loading Phase, you try to build up your normal fat stores by consuming as much fat as you can. When done well, it reduces the hunger you may feel when you enter the next phase.

Phase II is the very low calorie diet (VLCD), the phase that makes your friends raise their eyebrows when you tell them you're on a 500-calorie diet. However, the rest of the story is that hCG is causing anywhere from 1,500 to 4,000 calories a day to be released from your abnormal fat stores. Phase II ends two days after your last hCG dosage.

You continue on the 500-calorie diet those extra two days to allow time for all the hCG to be eliminated from your body. Phase II lasts between three and five weeks.

Phase III is called the maintenance phase. Careful attention to this phase helps your body stabilize itself at your new weight, reset its metabolism, and adjust to your lower appetite. The important restriction on Phase III is no starch, no sugar. If you do gain some weight, it should be no more than two pounds.

The Technique—Phase I Loading

There is something really weird about starting a diet by pigging out a few days first. I didn't know about Phase I when I first went to my naturopathic physician. In fact, I thought I had a jump start on the diet having just suffered through three days of the flu. Then to be told to eat basically as much as I could manage of high calorie, fat-dense foods for three days with the explanation that this was an important part of the diet—I felt like I had died and gone to heaven.

There are two basic approaches to Phase I. The first is to use the loading phase to eat the foods you will want to avoid on the diet—pizza, pasta dishes, cookies (my weakness), ice cream.

The better approach is to aim for healthy foods with a high fat content and avoid high sugar, high carb foods.

My experience: they both work. And believe it or not, I was ready to reduce my eating after two days of stuffing my face.

Phase I Loading summary: Start taking your hCG. Eat a lot.

The Technique—Phase II Very Low Calorie Diet (VLCD)

Here's the drill. Bear in mind, this is temporary. Only three to four weeks—your choice.

Take your hCG as directed by your medical provider. I took one sublingual tab first thing in the morning and last thing at night. My friend Emma gave herself one injection a day.

Breakfast:

Sorry, no eggs, hash brown, toast and jam. In fact, no food at all. This may take some getting used to, if you're a breakfast eater like me, but remember, it's only temporary.

What you can have is tea or coffee in any quantity without sugar. You may have only one tablespoonful of milk each day. Powder creamers are a no-no.

The only sweetener allowed is stevia, a natural, no-calorie sweetener.

Lunch:

Four ounces of veal, beef, chicken breast, fresh white fish, lobster, crab, or shrimp. Remove all visible fat and weigh the meat before cooking. It must be boiled or grilled without additional fat.

One type of vegetable only from the following: spinach, chard, chicory, beet-greens, green salad, tomatoes, celery, fennel, onions, red radishes, cucumbers, asparagus, cabbage. Never had fennel before? Now is your excuse to expand your dining repertoire.

One breadstick (called a grissino) or one Melba toast. Melba toast never tasted so good.

One serving of fruit: An apple or orange, a handful of strawberries, or one-half grapefruit. If you want, you can save the fruit and/or the Melba toast for a mid-afternoon snack. Or have it mid-morning to get you through to lunch.

Dinner:

The same four choices as lunch, except not the same choices. If you had chicken for lunch, you should have a different protein choice for dinner. Ditto for the vegetables and fruit.

Throughout the day, drink plenty of water. Aim for half your body weight in ounces.

Tea, coffee, plain water, mineral water are the only drinks allowed, but they may be taken in any quantity and at all times.

In addition, you are allowed the juice of one lemon (1 tablespoon) each day for cooking with or flavoring your water or tea.

Salt, pepper, vinegar, mustard powder, garlic, sweet basil, parsley, thyme, marjoram, and other herbs may be used for seasoning, but no oil, butter or salad dressing.

Read your labels. I was merrily using raspberry-flavored vinegar until I discovered it had as many calories as raspberry vinaigrette. On the other hand, my herb-flavored rice vinegar has zero calories.

The same holds true for bottled mineral or fizzy water. With all the types available these days, you want to find a brand with no flavoring and no artificial sweeteners. The good news is that you can buy flavored stevia and jazz it up yourself.

The traditional hCG diet plan allows for no more than 100 grams of protein per meal, twice a day. One hundred grams is equal to 3.52739 ounces. In the interest of simplicity, the Quick Start recipes call for 4 ounces. This way, you can buy a pound of ground beef and divide it into four equal portions. If you're not getting the results you want from the diet, you can always reduce your protein portions by 0.47261 ounces (I sometimes wonder if Dr. Simeons, being a metric guy, choose 100 grams because it was a nice round number).

Only low-intensity exercise is recommended during Phase II. A good goal is 30-60 minutes of walking every day, and you don't have to do it all at once. Since hCG remains in your system for about 48 hours after you take it, you continue on the VLCD eating plan for two days after your last dosage.

Phase II VLCD summary: Take your hCG. Eat no more than 500 calories a day. Walk. Stop taking hCG two days before the end of Phase II.

The Technique—Phase III Maintenance

The only restriction during Phase III is no starches, no sugar. In addition to breads and baked goods, the no-no list includes starchy vegetables such as potatoes, beans and corn. That's the bad news. The good news is that you can now eat more. You should not be hungry in Phase III.

You no longer need to weigh your food to get the proper portions. You do need to continue to weigh yourself.   The purpose of Phase III is to stabilize your weight loss and help you set a pattern for continuing to make healthy food choices.

You should stay on Phase III for the same length of time you were on Phase II.

You can also bump up the amount and intensity level of exercise if you are so inclined. If not, keep the walking going.

After the hCG Diet Quick Start: Your New Eating Plan

Your success in keeping off the weight you lost may require you to make some long-term changes in your eating and exercise patterns.

Here are four guidelines and one rule:

Guideline 1:   Enjoy how you feel at your new weight.   Become very conscious of how being thinner feels (great, huh?!).   The short-term enjoyment you may get out of eating something in some amount that you shouldn't is NOT WORTH jeopardizing that wonderful feeling.   Hold that thought.   And take the words "binge" and "overindulge" out of your vocabulary.   Not going there, not doing that anymore, no how, no way.

Guideline 2:   Remember what you practiced regarding portion control. You don't have to weigh your portions but you should have a better idea now of how much is enough, and stop there.

Guideline 3:   Slowly add new foods to your diet, keeping in mind portions and keeping a close eye on carbs in particular, like baked goods. While nothing is banned, you're just better off being very selective about what you put in your mouth and how often. For example, reintroduce bread to your diet one or days in the first week, just not every day. Be warned, however: you just may find you no longer crave baked goods if sugar is your downfall, or chips if you love your salt. I quit drinking diet pop altogether after my first round of hCG. It just wasn't appetizing anymore. The hCG diet has a wonderful cleansing effect on your body, and after weeks of healthy, fresh food, you may find it quite easy to pass on high fat, oversauced, oversweetened, overfried, oversalted foods. This is good, and good for you.

Guideline 4: Keep moving! Make physical activity of some kind a daily priority.

The One-and-Only-Rule: Weigh Yourself Every Day. Make your scale your friend. Yes, it's possible. I still can't quite believe mine, which delights me no end.

And that's the skinny on hCG.

Chapter Two: The hCG Diet Quick Start Approach

Remember my friend Emma who thoroughly researched the diet before taking the plunge? If you're like Emma, there's plenty more information on hCG online to answer all your questions.

But if you're like me, once you decide to do something, you're in a hurry to get started.

First Things First

Make an appointment with a medical provider. Your medical provider will discuss your weight loss goals with you, help you decide if the hCG diet is a good fit for you, do a body composition analysis as a benchmark, and discuss the different options for taking hCG. Your medical provider can also give you access to pharmacy quality hCG. It may be cheaper through other sources such as websites or your local box store, but the quality can't be guaranteed. In short, if you're going to do it, do it right. Back to your options: My friend Emma opted for self-administered injections, but then, she's a nurse. I had excellent results using sublingual (under the tongue) tabs or pills. We both received our hCG from naturopathic physicians. hCG is also available in a liquid form (drops).

Plan when to start. One of the beauties of this diet is the very low calorie diet (Phase I) is fairly short. It may not feel like it when you're in the middle of it, but it's much faster than any other program I've tried. So, take a look at your calendar and pick your block of time when you don't have food-centric social events.

Get rid of temptations in your cupboards. Set up your kitchen to support your diet goals as best you can. Naturally, if you don't live alone, this may not be entirely possible. In that case, ask for cooperation and get creative.

Buy a small kitchen scale. Yes, you will be weighing your food to control your portions.

Scan through the hCG Diet Quick Start Cookbook. It's designed to do the hard work of meal planning. And to send you to the supermarket with a list of what to have on hand and what to buy for that week.

Getting a new diet usually means learning new recipes, and the hCG Diet Quick Start Cookbook is no exception. The good news is that we've kept the recipes easy and simple with an emphasis on taste appeal. Better yet, you cook something once and eat it twice. Yes—leftovers! None of this single-serving-recipe business. Leftovers are convenient, toteable, quick, and brainless. Quick Start leftovers are tasty too.

Off to a Quick Start

Here's what's coming, all geared to take out the guesswork and decision making out of your hCG diet.

Your list of kitchen staples

Four one-week menus for Phase II Very Low Calorie Diet (VLCD)

These menus are labeled A through D.

The menus feature a variety of proteins. Week A contains chicken, beef, and seafood recipes. Week B contains chicken, beef, and vegetarian recipes. Week C is beef-less, and contains chicken, seafood, and vegetarian recipes. Finally, Week D features only vegetarian recipes.

Each menu for a given day complies with the hCG diet calorie restrictions—no calorie counting required!

The idea for your "quick start" is that you only have to decide which week or weeks of recipes you want to follow. You don't have to do all of them. You can repeat one menu, like the Week D vegetarian menu, for the entire course of your Phase II VLCD.

Each week contains your complete shopping list.
If you've stocked your pantry with your staples, one trip to the store each week and you're good to go!

Four one-week menus for Phase III Maintenance
These menus are labeled E through H.

The proteins in Weeks E through H match those in Phase II VLCD weeks A through D. So if you prefer not to eat beef, you can choose between Weeks C and D of Phase II and Weeks G and H of Phase III. And of course each week sends you to the store with your shopping list.

I think I'm a smart cookie, but I'm a lazy cook. The hardest part of cooking for me has always been menu planning and being sure I have on hand what I need so I don't have to do creative substituting. If you're like me, the hCG Diet Quick Start Cookbook was expressly designed for you.

Are you ready? Good luck and here's to looking at a thinner new you!

Chapter Three: List of Staples for the hCG Diet Quick Start

Here is your list of staples or basics. Use it to check on the current state of your pantry and see what you need to pick up from the grocery store.

This may seem like a long list but it's not when you consider you're outfitting your kitchen for weeks to come. Plus all the staples on this list are basics for many other recipes and most will keep well.

Coffee
Tea
Bottled water (fizzy water, meaning carbonated water, is fine but read your label to be sure no sweetener added)

Breadsticks and/or Melba toast
Sea or kosher salt
Ground pepper or peppercorns

Low-sodium beef, chicken and/or vegetable broth
Fresh garlic
Tomato paste
Tomato sauce
Dried cranberries
Almond extract

Stevia packets (the only sweetener allowed for Phase II; becoming more available in grocery stores but check your local health food store if you can't find it)
Agave nectar (ditto regarding availability)

Red wine vinegar
White wine vinegar
Apple cider vinegar
Balsamic vinegar
Rice vinegar, plain
Tarragon vinegar

A word about vinegars: I grew up with two—apple cider vinegar and white vinegar. Since then I've discovered the wonderful flavors of different types of vinegar. These are all good basics to have on hand as you explore new tastes.

Olive oil

Bragg's Liquid Aminos (similar to soy sauce; look for in your health food store)
Worcestershire sauce
Low-sodium soy sauce
Prepared mustard
Sugar-free ketchup
Hot sauce (Tabasco)

Dried herbs and spices (Group One):
Onion flakes
Garlic granules
Chili powder
Paprika
Cinnamon
Ground nutmeg
Oregano

Basil
Parsley

Dried herbs and spices (Group Two):
Cumin
Cayenne pepper
Red pepper flakes
Bay leaf
Thyme
Dried mustard
Poppy seeds
Sesame seeds
Cardamom
Curry powder
Coriander
Turmeric
Rubbed Sage
Ground allspice
Old Bay seasoning
Creole seasoning
Herbs de Provence

A word about spices and herbs: I love the spices, available in bulk, from my local health food store. I can buy as much or as little as I want and the freshness and quality are unbeatable. The first list above includes the more commonly used seasonings. The second list has seasonings either used less frequently or in small quantities.

Chapter Four: Quick Start Menus for Phase II VLCD

Want handy printer-ready menus for posting on your refrigerator? See the Appendix.

The menus for the starred dishes are in Chapter Eight.

Week A Menu featuring Chicken, Beef, and Seafood

Day 1 (495 calories)

Breakfast
   Coffee, tea, or water
Lunch
   **Super Beef Chili (194 calories)
   Breadstick or Melba Toast
Dinner
   **Chicken with Orange and Fresh Basil (216 calories)
   Lettuce Salad (2 cups)
Snack
   Strawberries (10 medium)
   Breadstick or Melba Toast

Day 2 (491 calories)

Breakfast
   Coffee, tea, or water
Lunch
   **Chicken with Orange and Fresh Basil (216 calories)

Asparagus, steamed (2 cups)
Breadstick or Melba Toast

Dinner
**Tilapia with Strawberry Salsa (160 calories)
Spinach, steamed (3 cups raw)

Snack
Breadstick or Melba Toast

Day 3 (504 calories)

Breakfast
Coffee, tea, or water

Lunch
**Super Beef Chili (194 calories)
Breadstick or Melba Toast

Dinner
**Tilapia with Strawberry Salsa (160 calories)
Lettuce Salad (2 cups)

Snack
Apple
Breadstick or Melba Toast

Day 4 (501 calories)

Breakfast
Coffee, tea, or water

Lunch
**Chinese Orange Beef Stir Fry (254 calories)

Dinner
**Easy Chicken Cacciatore (175 calories)
Breadstick or Melba Toast

Snack
Strawberries (10 medium)
Breadstick or Melba Toast

Day 5 (501 calories)

Breakfast
Coffee, tea, or water

Lunch
  **Easy Chicken Cacciatore (175 calories)
  Breadstick or Melba Toast
Dinner
  **Chinese Orange Beef Stir Fry (254 calories)
Snack
  1/2 Grapefruit

Day 6 (504 calories)

Breakfast
  Coffee, tea, or water
Lunch
  **Tangy Apple Slaw (134 calories)
  Grilled Chicken Breast (4 oz.)
Dinner
  **Broiled Lemon Garlic Shrimp (120 calories)
  Lettuce Salad (2 cups)
  Breadstick or Melba Toast
Snack
  Orange
  Breadstick or Melba Toast

Day 7 (503 calories)

Breakfast
  Coffee, tea, or water
Lunch
  **Broiled Lemon Garlic Shrimp (120 calories)
  Spinach Salad (3 cups)
  Breadstick or Melba Toast
Dinner
  **The Big Bodacious Burger (158 calories)
  **Tangy Apple Slaw (134 calories)
Snack
  ½ Grapefruit
  Breadstick or Melba Toast

Week B Menu featuring Chicken, Beef, and Vegetarian

Day 1 (500 calories)

Breakfast
   Coffee, tea, or water
Lunch
   **Cream of Fennel Soup (120 calories)
   1/2 cup nonfat cottage cheese
   Breadstick or Melba Toast
Dinner
   **Tuscan Bistecca with Lemon (220 calories)
   Lettuce Salad (2 cups)
Snack
   Strawberries (10 medium)
   Breadstick or Melba Toast

Day 2 (502 calories)

Breakfast
   Coffee, tea, or water
Lunch
   **Easy Onion Frittata (215 calories)
   Breadstick or Melba Toast
Dinner
   **Wrapped Up Chicken Fajitas (180 calories)
   Served with Lettuce for Wrapping
Snack
   1/2 Grapefruit
   Breadstick or Melba Toast

Day 3 (506 calories)

Breakfast
   Coffee, tea, or water
Lunch
   **Tuscan Bistecca with Lemon (220 calories)
   Sliced over Spinach Salad (3 cups)

Dinner
   **Easy Onion Frittata (215 calories)
Snack
   Strawberries (10 medium)
   Breadstick or Melba Toast

Day 4 (478 calories)

Breakfast
   Coffee, tea, or water
Lunch
   **Wrapped Up Chicken Fajitas (180 calories)
   Served over Lettuce Salad (2 cups)
   Breadstick or Melba Toast
Dinner
   **Sweet Strawberry Souffle Omelet (170 calories)
   Spinach Salad (3 cups)
Snack
   1/2 Grapefruit
   Breadstick or Melba Toast

Day 5 (500 calories)

Breakfast
   Coffee, tea, or water
Lunch
   **Cream of Fennel Soup (120 calories)
   1/2 cup nonfat cottage cheese
Dinner
   **Skewered Steak and Red Onions (235 calories)
   Breadstick or Melba Toast
Snack
   Strawberries (10 medium)
   Breadstick or Melba Toast

Day 6 (499 calories)

Breakfast
   Coffee, tea, or water

Lunch
    **Tomato Bruschetta Omelet (155 calories)
    Breadstick or Melba Toast
Dinner
    **Savory Sage and Apple Chicken Burgers (180 calories)
    Steamed Asparagus (2 cups)
Snack
    Orange
    Breadstick or Melba Toast

Day 7 (500 calories)

Breakfast
    Coffee, tea, or water
Lunch
    **Savory Sage and Apple Chicken Burgers (180 calories)
    Served with Lettuce for Wrapping
Dinner
    **Skewered Steak and Red Onions (235 calories)
    Breadstick or Melba Toast
Snack
    Strawberries (10 medium)
    Breadstick or Melba Toast

Week C Menu featuring Chicken, Seafood, and Vegetarian

Day 1 (497 calories)

Breakfast
    Coffee, tea, or water
Lunch
    **French Onion Soup (120 calories)
    1/2 cup nonfat cottage cheese
    1/2 Apple

Dinner
  **Herb Roasted Chicken with Lemon and Fennel
  (187 calories)
  Breadstick or Melba Toast
Snack
  Strawberries (10 medium)
  Breadstick or Melba Toast

Day 2 (499 calories)

Breakfast
  Coffee, tea, or water
Lunch
  **Herb Roasted Chicken with Lemon and Fennel
  (187 calories)
  Breadstick or Melba Toast
Dinner
  **Orange Soy Glazed Shrimp (227 calories)
  Lettuce Salad (2 cups)
Snack
  Strawberries (10 medium)
  Breadstick or Melba Toast

Day 3 (496 calories)

Breakfast
  Coffee, tea, or water
Lunch
  **Orange Soy Glazed Shrimp (227 calories)
  Cucumber Spears (2 cups)
  Breadstick or Melba Toast
Dinner
  **Spinach Soy Patties with Lemon Sauce Glaze
  (125 calories)
  Spinach Salad (1 ½ cups)
Snack
  1/2 Grapefruit
  Breadstick or Melba Toast

Day 4 (505 calories)

Breakfast
Coffee, tea, or water
Lunch
**Spinach Soy Patties with Lemon Sauce Glaze
(125 calories)
Spinach Salad (1 ½ cups)
Breadstick or Melba Toast
Dinner
**Asian Chicken Roll Ups (200 calories)
1/2 Orange
Snack
Apple
Breadstick or Melba Toast

Day 5 (503 calories)

Breakfast
Coffee, tea, or water
Lunch
**Asian Chicken Roll Ups (200 calories)
1/2 Orange
Dinner
**So-y Delicious Chili (133 calories)
Breadstick or Melba Toast
Snack
Apple
Breadstick or Melba Toast

Day 6 (503 calories)

Breakfast
Coffee, tea, or water
Lunch
**French Onion Soup (120 calories)
1/2 cup nonfat cottage cheese
1/2 Apple

Dinner
   **Petit Baked Crab Cakes (158 calories)
   Lettuce Salad (2 cups)
Snack
   Orange
   Breadstick or Melba

Day 7 (486 calories)

Breakfast
   Coffee, tea, or water
Lunch
   **Petit Baked Crab Cakes (158 calories)
   Spinach Salad (3 cups)
Dinner
   **Apple Cottage Cheese Dip (222 calories)
   Breadstick or Melba Toast
Snack
   ½ Grapefruit

Week D Menu featuring Vegetarian

Day 1 (488 calories)

Breakfast
   Coffee, tea, or water
Lunch
   **Minty Radish and Grapefruit Slaw (145 calories)
   1/2 cup nonfat cottage cheese
Dinner
   **So-y Delicious Chili (133 calories)
   Breadstick or Melba Toast
Snack
   Apple
   Breadstick or Melba Toast

Day 2 (459 calories)

Breakfast
   Coffee, tea, or water

Lunch
   **So-y Delicious Chili (133 calories)
   Breadstick or Melba Toast
Dinner
   **Sweet Strawberry Souffle Omelet (170 calories)
   Spinach Salad (3 cups)
Snack
   Apple
   Breadstick or Melba Toast

Day 3 (487 calories)

Breakfast
   Coffee, tea, or water
Lunch
   **Apple Cottage Cheese Dip (222 calories)
Dinner
   **Tomato Bruschetta Omelet (155 calories)
   Breadstick or Melba Toast
Snack
   Orange
   Breadstick or Melba Toast

Day 4 (454 calories)

Breakfast
   Coffee, tea, or water
Lunch
   **Tangy Apple Slaw (134 calories)
   1/2 cup nonfat cottage cheese
Dinner
   **Spinach Soy Patties with Lemon Sauce Glaze
   (125 calories)
   Spinach Salad (1 ½ cups)
   Breadstick or Melba Toast
Snack
   Orange
   Breadstick or Melba Toast

Day 5 (486 calories)

Breakfast
Coffee, tea, or water
Lunch
**Spinach Soy Patties with Lemon Sauce Glaze (125 calories)
Spinach Salad (1 ½ cups)
Dinner
**Easy Onion Frittata (215 calories)
Breadstick or Melba Toast
Snack
Apple
Breadstick or Melba Toast

Day 6 (464 calories)

Breakfast
Coffee, tea, or water
Lunch
**Tangy Apple Slaw (134 calories)
1/2 cup nonfat cottage cheese
Dinner
**Easy Onion Frittata (215 calories)
Breadstick or Melba Toast
Snack
Breadstick or Melba Toast

Day 7 (471 calories)

Breakfast
Coffee, tea, or water
Lunch
**Cucumber and Orange Salad (115 calories)
1/2 cup nonfat cottage cheese
Breadstick or Melba Toast
Dinner
Grilled Soy Patty
Spinach Salad (3 cups)

Snack
  Apple
  Breadstick or Melba Toast

Chapter Five: Quick Start Shopping Lists for Phase II VLCD

Want a handy printer-ready checklist for your weekly shopping? See the Appendix.

Shopping List for Week A Menu (Chicken/Beef/Seafood)

Protein:
12 oz. lean ground beef (95%)
8 oz. lean beef steak, such as tenderloin
1 lb. boneless, skinless chicken breasts
8 oz. frozen uncooked large shrimp
8 oz. tilapia fillets, fresh or frozen
Vegetables:
8 oz. asparagus
4 medium tomatoes
Lettuce greens (to equal 6 cups)
Raw spinach, regular or baby (to equal 6 cups)
1 large Napa cabbage
Fresh basil, parsley, and mint
Fruit:
5 medium oranges
Lemons (at least 2)
1 medium grapefruit
2 x 16 oz. boxes fresh strawberries
3 medium apples

Shopping List for Week B Menu (Chicken/Beef/Vegetarian)

Protein:
8 oz. lean beef steak, such as tenderloin
8 oz. boneless, skinless chicken breasts
8 oz. ground chicken breast
Large eggs, 18 count package
8 oz. (1 cup) nonfat cottage cheese
Vegetables:
8 oz. asparagus
1 medium tomato
Lettuce greens (to equal 8 cups)
Raw spinach, regular or baby (to equal 9 cups)
1 large fennel bulb
2 medium yellow onions
2 medium red onions
Fruit:
5 medium oranges
Lemons (at least 2)
1 medium grapefruit
2 x 16 oz. boxes fresh strawberries
2 medium apples

Shopping List for Week C Menu (Chicken/Seafood/Vegetarian)

Protein:
8 oz. boneless, skinless chicken breasts
8 oz. ground chicken breast
8 oz. frozen uncooked large shrimp
8 oz. lump crab meat
8 oz. plain soy patties
12 oz. nonfat cottage cheese
Vegetables:
Celery stalks (2 cups)
1 large cucumber
Lettuce greens (to equal 4 cups)
Raw spinach, regular or baby (to equal 9 cups)

1 large fennel bulb
2 medium yellow onions
Small knob fresh ginger
Fruit:
5 medium oranges
Lemons (at least 3)
1 medium grapefruit
1 16 oz. box fresh strawberries
4 medium apples

Shopping List for Week D Menu (Vegetarian)

Protein:
20 oz. plain soy patties
20 oz. (2 ½ cups) nonfat cottage cheese
Large eggs 16
Vegetables:
Celery stalks (2 cups)
1 large cucumber
Raw spinach, regular or baby (to equal 12 cups)
Red radishes (2 cups)
2 medium yellow onions
3 medium tomatoes
Small white or Napa cabbage
Fruit:
4 medium oranges
Lemons (at least 4)
1 medium grapefruit
1 8 oz. box fresh strawberries
7 medium apples

Chapter Six: Quick Start Menus for Phase III Maintenance

Want handy printer-ready menus for posting on your refrigerator? See the Appendix.

The menus for the starred dishes are in Chapter Nine.

Week E Menu featuring Chicken, Beef, and Seafood

Each day has 1400 to 1700 calories

Day 1

Breakfast
   Two eggs scrambled
   Turkey bacon
   1 orange
   Coffee or tea
Snack
   Sugar-free yogurt
Lunch
   **Creamy Chicken Chowder (272 calories)
   Celery and bell pepper strips
Snack
   Apricot halves with cottage cheese
Dinner
   Grilled sirloin steak
   Asparagus spears
   Lettuce wedge with light salad dressing

Snack/Dessert
  **Apple Crumb Pie (177 calories)

Day 2

Breakfast
  Two egg spinach omelet
  Coffee or tea
Snack
  Sugar-free yogurt
Lunch
  Grilled turkey burger
  Sliced tomato and sautéed onion
Snack
  Swiss cheese wedge
  Apple
Dinner
  **Sensational Salmon Burger (214 calories)
  Sautéed green beans
  Lettuce salad with light dressing
Snack/Dessert
  **Coconut Macaroons (59 calories) with glass of
  Almond or soy milk

Day 3

Breakfast
  Poached eggs with turkey sausage
  Orange
  Coffee or tea
Snack
  Cottage cheese with
  Apple and cinnamon
Lunch
  **Primavera Salad (221 calories)
  Sliced grilled chicken breast
  Pineapple chunks
Snack
  Sugar-free yogurt

Dinner
  **Hearty Beef Stroganoff (260 calories)
  Lettuce salad with light dressing
Snack/Dessert
  **Apple Crumb Pie (177 calories)

Day 4

Breakfast
  **Nutty Orange Scones (250 calories)
  ½ grapefruit
  Coffee or tea
Snack
  Sugar-free yogurt
Lunch
  **Creamy Chicken Chowder (272 calories)
  **Primavera Salad (221 calories)
Snack
  Apricot halves with cottage cheese
Dinner
  **Sensational Salmon Burger (214 calories)
  Sautéed green beans
  Spinach salad with light dressing
Snack/Dessert
  **Coconut Macaroons (59 calories) with glass of
  Almond or soymilk

Day 5

Breakfast
  Two eggs scrambled
  Cottage cheese
  Orange
  Coffee or tea
Snack
  Sugar-free yogurt
Lunch
  Chef's salad with lettuce, roast beef, and
  Swiss cheese, tomato, carrot, cucumber and
  Light dressing

Snack
    **Nutty Orange Scones (250 calories) with glass of
    Almond or soymilk
Dinner
    **Moroccan Chicken Breasts (440 calories)
    Asparagus spears
Snack/Dessert
    **Coconut Macaroons (59 calories)
    Pineapple chunks

Day 6

Breakfast
    Poached eggs with turkey sausage
    ½ grapefruit
    Coffee or tea
Snack
    Plain yogurt with
    Apple and cinnamon
Lunch
    **Primavera Salad (221 calories)
    Sliced grilled chicken breast
    Apricot halves
Snack
    Swiss cheese wedge
    Orange
Dinner
    **Hearty Beef Stroganoff (260 calories)
    Lettuce salad with light dressing
Snack/Dessert
    **Coconut Macaroons (59 calories) with glass
    Almond or Soymilk

Day 7

Breakfast
    **Nutty Orange Scones (250 calories)
    Cottage cheese
    Coffee or tea
Snack

Sugar-free yogurt
Lunch
   Turkey burger
   Sliced tomato and lettuce
   Apple
Snack
   Orange
Dinner
   **Moroccan Chicken Breasts (440 calories)
   Lettuce salad with light dressing
Snack/Dessert
   **Coconut Macaroons (59 calories)
   Pineapple chunks

Week F Menu featuring Chicken, Beef, and Vegetarian

Each day has 1400 to 1700 calories

Day 1

Breakfast
   Two eggs scrambled
   Turkey bacon
   1 orange
   Coffee or tea
Snack
   Sugar-free yogurt
Lunch
   **Creamy Broccoli Soup (107 calories)
   Lettuce salad with light dressing and
   Sliced turkey breast
Snack
   Apricot halves with cottage cheese
Dinner
   **Tangy Stuffed Peppers (282 calories)
   Lettuce wedge with light salad dressing

Snack/Dessert
  **Apple Crumb Pie (177 calories)

Day 2

Breakfast
  Two egg spinach omelet
  ½ grapefruit
  Coffee or tea
Snack
  Sugar-free yogurt
Lunch
  **Tangy Stuffed Peppers (282 calories)
  Spinach salad with light salad dressing
Snack
  Cheddar cheese wedge
  Apple
Dinner
  **Quick and Easy Chicken Stew (253 calories)
  Lettuce salad with light dressing
Snack/Dessert
  **Grilled Peach Parfait (117 calories)

Day 3

Breakfast
  **Crustless Quiche with Sun Dried Tomatoes (125
  calories)
  Orange
  Coffee or tea
Snack
  Cottage cheese with
  Pineapple chunks
Lunch
  Sliced grilled chicken breast
  **Guacamole (91 calories)
  Celery and bell pepper for dipping
Snack
  Sugar-free yogurt

Dinner
   **Teriyaki Beef with Snow Peas (351 calories)
Snack/Dessert
   **Apple Crumb Pie (177 calories)

Day 4

Breakfast
   Veggie omelet with cheddar cheese
   ½ grapefruit
   Coffee or tea
Snack
   Sugar-free yogurt
Lunch
   **Creamy Broccoli Soup (107 calories)
   Spinach salad with light dressing and
   Sliced turkey breast
Snack
   **Guacamole (91 calories)
   Celery and bell pepper for dipping
Dinner
   **Pork Chops with Apples and Kraut (330 calories)
   Sautéed green beans
Snack/Dessert
   **Grilled Peach Parfait (117 calories)

Day 5

Breakfast
   **Crustless Quiche with Sun Dried Tomatoes (125 calories)
   Orange
   Coffee or tea
Snack
   Sugar-free yogurt
Lunch
   **Teriyaki Beef with Snow Peas (351 calories)
   Pineapple chunks

Snack
  Apple
  Cheddar cheese
Dinner
  **Super Juicy Roast Lemon Chicken (367 calories)
  Lettuce salad with light dressing
Snack/Dessert
  **Coconut Macaroons (59 calories) with glass of Almond or soymilk

Day 6

Breakfast
  Poached eggs with turkey sausage
  ½ grapefruit
  Coffee or tea
Snack
  Sugar-free yogurt
Lunch
  **Super Juicy Roast Lemon Chicken (367 calories)
  Spinach salad with light dressing
Snack
  Orange
Dinner
  **Pork Chops with Apples and Kraut (330 calories)
  Sautéed green beans
Snack/Dessert
  **Nutty Orange Scones (250 calories)

Day 7

Breakfast
  **Crustless Quiche with Sun Dried Tomatoes (125 calories)
  ½ grapefruit
  Coffee or tea

Snack
　Sugar-free yogurt
Lunch
　**Creamy Broccoli Soup (107 calories)
　Lettuce salad with light dressing and
　Sliced turkey breast
Snack
　Orange
Dinner
　**Tangy Stuffed Peppers (282 calories)
　Spinach salad with light salad dressing
　Apple
Snack/Dessert
　**Coconut Macaroons (59 calories)
　Pineapple chunks

Week G Menu featuring Chicken, Seafood, and Vegetarian

Each day has 1400 to 1700 calories

Day 1

Breakfast
　Two eggs scrambled
　Turkey bacon
　1 orange
　Coffee or tea
Snack
　Sugar-free yogurt
Lunch
　**Creamy Chicken Chowder (272 calories)
　Lettuce salad with light dressing
Snack
　Apricot halves with cottage cheese
Dinner
**Super Shrimp Gumbo (173 calories)
　Lettuce wedge with light salad dressing

Snack/Dessert
 **Apple Crumb Pie (177 calories) with glass of
 Almond or soymilk

Day 2

Breakfast
 Two egg spinach omelet
 ½ grapefruit
 Coffee or tea
Snack
 Sugar-free yogurt
Lunch
 **Super Shrimp Gumbo (173 calories)
 Spinach salad with light salad dressing
Snack
 Muenster cheese wedge
 Apple
Dinner
 **Terrific Turkey Loaf (240 calories)
 Steamed broccoli
 Lettuce salad with light dressing
Snack/Dessert
 **Favorite Fruit Sorbet (30 calories)
 **Coconut Macaroons (59 calories)

Day 3

Breakfast
 **Crustless Quiche with Sun Dried Tomatoes (125
 calories)
 Orange
 Coffee or tea
Snack
 Cottage cheese with
 Pineapple chunks
Lunch
 **Terrific Turkey Loaf (240 calories)
 Carrot sticks
 Lettuce salad with light dressing

Snack
   Sugar-free yogurt
Dinner
   **Seared Ahi Tuna with Wasabi Dressing (203 calories)
   Steamed broccoli
Snack/Dessert
   **Apple Crumb Pie (177 calories) with glass of Almond or soymilk

Day 4

Breakfast
   Veggie omelet
   Turkey bacon
   ½ grapefruit
   Coffee or tea
Snack
   Sugar-free yogurt
Lunch
   **Creamy Chicken Chowder (272 calories)
   Spinach salad with light dressing
Snack
   Muenster cheese wedge
   Apple
Dinner
   **Lemon-Lime Fish Fillet with Salsa (330 calories)
   Sautéed green beans
Snack/Dessert
   **Favorite Fruit Sorbet (30 calories)
   **Coconut Macaroons (59 calories)

Day 5

Breakfast
   2 eggs scrambled
   Turkey bacon
   Orange
   Coffee or tea

Snack
  Sugar-free yogurt
Lunch
  **Seared Ahi Tuna with Wasabi Dressing (203 *calories*)
  Steamed broccoli
  Pineapple chunks
Snack
  Apple
  Cottage cheese
Dinner
  **Terrific Turkey Loaf (240 calories)
  Steamed broccoli
  Lettuce salad with light dressing
Snack/Dessert
  **Nutty Orange Scones (250 calories)

Day 6

Breakfast
  Poached eggs
  ½ grapefruit
  Coffee or tea
Snack
  Sugar-free yogurt
Lunch
  **Lemon-Lime Fish Fillet with Salsa (330 calories)
  Spinach salad with light dressing
Snack
  Orange
Dinner
  **Super Shrimp Gumbo (173 calories)
  Sautéed green beans
Snack/Dessert
  **Favorite Fruit Sorbet (30 calories)
  **Coconut Macaroons (59 calories)

Day 7

Breakfast
    **Nutty Orange Scones (250 calories)
    ½ grapefruit
    Coffee or tea
Snack
    Sugar-free yogurt
Lunch
    **Super Shrimp Gumbo (173 calories)
    Spinach salad with light dressing
Snack
    Orange
Dinner
    **Terrific Turkey Loaf (240 calories)
    Steamed broccoli
    Lettuce salad with light dressing
    Apple
Snack/Dessert
    **Coconut Macaroons (59 calories)
    Pineapple chunks

Week H Menu featuring Vegetarian

Each day has 1400 to 1700 calories

Day 1

Breakfast
    Two eggs scrambled
    1 orange
    Coffee or tea
Snack
    Sugar-free yogurt
Lunch
    **Creamy Broccoli Soup (107 calories)
    **Nutty Orange Scones (250 calories)
    Lettuce salad with light dressing

Snack
  Apricot halves with cottage cheese
Dinner
  **Herbed Portobello Burger (154 calories)
  Slice American cheese
  Sauteed onions
  Sliced tomatoes
  Lettuce wedge with light salad dressing
Snack/Dessert
  **Apple Crumb Pie (177 calories)* with glass of
  Almond or soymilk

Day 2

Breakfast
  Two egg spinach omelet
  ½ grapefruit
  Coffee or tea
Snack
  Sugar-free yogurt
Lunch
  **Eggplant Rollatini (374 calories)
  Spinach salad with light salad dressing
Snack
  Orange
  Apple
Dinner
  **Indonesian Vegetarian Stew (457 calories)
Snack/Dessert
  **Favorite Fruit Sorbet (30 calories)
  **Coconut Macaroons (59 calories)

Day 3

Breakfast
  **Crustless Quiche with Sun Dried Tomatoes (125
  calories)
  Orange
  Coffee or tea

Snack
  Cottage cheese with
  Pineapple chunks
Lunch
  **Indonesian Vegetarian Stew (457 calories)
Snack
  Sugar-free yogurt
Dinner
  **Primavera Salad (221 calories)
  ^^Nutty Orange Scones (250 calories)
  Apricot halves
Snack/Dessert
  **Apple Crumb Pie (177 calories) with glass of
  Almond or soymilk

Day 4

Breakfast
  Veggie omelet with cheese
  ½ grapefruit
  Coffee or tea
Snack
  Sugar-free yogurt
Lunch
  **Creamy Broccoli Soup (107 calories)
  **Nutty Orange Scones (250 calories)
  Lettuce salad with light dressing
Snack
  Cottage cheese
  Apple
Dinner
  **Eggplant Rollatini (374 calories)
  Spinach salad with light salad dressing
Snack/Dessert
  **Favorite Fruit Sorbet (30 calories)
  **Coconut Macaroons (59 calories)

Day 5

Breakfast
   **Nutty Orange Scones (250 calories)
   ½ grapefruit
   Coffee or tea
Snack
   Sugar-free yogurt
Lunch
   **Primavera Salad (221 calories)
   Apricot halves
Snack
   **Guacamole (91 calories)
   Red bell pepper strips
Dinner
   **Crustless Quiche with Sun Dried Tomatoes (125 calories)
   Steamed broccoli
   Lettuce salad with light dressing
Snack/Dessert
   Apple
   Cottage cheese

Day 6

Breakfast
   Poached eggs
   ½ grapefruit
   Coffee or tea
Snack
   Sugar-free yogurt
Lunch
   **Guacamole (91 calories)
   American cheese slice
   Celery sticks
   Spinach salad with light dressing
Snack
   Orange

Dinner
   **Indonesian Vegetarian Stew (457 calories)
Snack/Dessert
   **Favorite Fruit Sorbet (30 calories)
   **Coconut Macaroons (59 calories)

Day 7

Breakfast
   **Nutty Orange Scones (250 calories)
   ½ grapefruit
   Coffee or tea
Snack
   Sugar-free yogurt
Lunch
   **Creamy Broccoli Soup (107 calories)
   Cottage cheese
   Spinach salad with light dressing
Snack
   Orange
   Pineapple chunks
Dinner
   **Herbed Portobello Burger (154 calories)
   Slice American cheese
   Sauteed onions
   Sliced tomatoes
   Lettuce wedge with light salad dressing
Snack/Dessert
   **Coconut Macaroons (59 calories) with glass of
   Almond or soymilk

Chapter Seven: Quick Start Shopping Lists for Phase III Maintenance

Shopping List for Week E Menu (Chicken/Beef/Seafood)

Protein:
1 x 4oz. sirloin steak
1 lb. beef round steak
2 split chicken breasts
1 lb. boneless, skinless chicken breasts
8 oz. ground turkey
8 oz. salmon fillet
1 dozen large eggs
Turkey bacon
Turkey breakfast sausage
3 oz. deli roast beef

Dairy:
1 pt. lowfat cottage cheese
3 oz. Swiss cheese
4 oz. mozzarella cheese
Unsweetened almond milk or soymilk
1 pt. plain yogurt
3 small sugar-free yogurts
Unsalted butter

Vegetables:
2 medium tomatoes
Grape tomatoes
Lettuce greens (to equal 8 cups)
Raw spinach, regular or baby (to equal 4 cups)
3 medium yellow onions

1 small red onion
10 oz. white mushrooms
Medium cucumber
Broccoli florets
Shredded carrots
Celery sticks
2 medium red bell peppers
1 lb. asparagus, fresh or frozen
1 lb. green beans, fresh or frozen
Fresh basil, dill, and cilantro
Fruit:
5 medium oranges
Lemons (at least 1)
1 grapefruit
1 cup fresh pineapple
2 Granny Smith apples
4 eating apples
Small box prunes
Medium can apricot halves, no-added-sugar
Small unsweetened applesauce
Other:
Almond flour
Unsweetened shredded coconut

Shopping List for Week F Menu (Chicken/Beef/Vegetarian)

Protein:
8 oz. beef sirloin or tenderloin steak
1 lb. ground beef or veal
4 chicken leg quarters
1 lb. boneless, skinless chicken breasts
1 lb. thin loin or rib pork chops
1 dozen large eggs
Turkey bacon
Turkey breakfast sausage
8 oz. deli sliced turkey breast
Dairy:
1 pt. lowfat cottage cheese

3 oz. cheddar cheese
Unsweetened almond milk, soymilk, or cow's milk
6 small sugar-free yogurts
Vegetables:
1 medium tomato
Lettuce greens (to equal 10 cups)
Raw spinach, regular or baby (to equal 8 cups)
3 medium yellow onions
1 medium avocado
1 bunch scallions
1 ½ lb. broccoli
Small bag whole carrots
Celery sticks
1 medium red bell pepper
2 large green bell peppers
4 oz. snow peas
1 lb. green beans, fresh or frozen
Fresh rosemary and parsley
1 x 15 oz. can sauerkraut
Fruit:
5 medium oranges
Lemons (at least 2)
1 lime
2 grapefruit
1 ½ cup fresh pineapple
1 large peach
2 Granny Smith apples
4 eating apples
Small can apricot halves, no-added-sugar

Shopping List for Week G Menu (Chicken/Seafood/Vegetarian)

Protein:
1 lb. ground turkey
8 oz boneless, skinless chicken breasts
1 lb. medium shrimp
8 oz. ahi tuna
8 oz. cod or scrod

1 dozen large eggs
Turkey bacon
Dairy:
8 oz. lowfat cottage cheese
3 oz. Muenster cheese
Unsweetened almond milk, soymilk, or cow's milk
6 small sugar-free yogurts
Vegetables:
Lettuce greens (to equal 8 cups)
Raw spinach, regular or baby (to equal 7 cups)
Watercress (2 cups)
2 medium yellow onions
8 oz. broccoli
Celery sticks
1 medium red bell pepper
1 medium green bell pepper
8 oz. green beans, fresh or frozen
5 medium oranges
Fruit:
1 Lemon
1 lime
2 grapefruit
½ cup fresh pineapple
2 Granny Smith apples
2 eating apples
Small can apricot halves, no-added-sugar
Choice of fruit for sorbet
Other:
 Ground flaxseed
Wasabi powder

Shopping List for Week H Menu (Vegetarian)

Protein:
1 dozen large eggs
8 oz. extra firm tofu
Dairy:
2 pts. lowfat cottage cheese

4 oz. American cheese
Unsweetened almond milk, soymilk, or cow's milk
6 small sugar-free yogurts
Vegetables:
Lettuce greens (to equal 8 cups)
Raw spinach, regular or baby (to equal 10 cups)
3 medium yellow onions
2 lb. broccoli
1 medium red bell pepper
1 medium avocado
2 large Portobello mushrooms
1 large eggplant
4 oz. cauliflower
4 oz. green beans, fresh or frozen
1 jar marinara sauce, no-sugar-added
Fruit:
5 medium oranges
1 lime
3 grapefruit
1 cup fresh pineapple
2 Granny Smith apples
3 eating apples
Large can apricot halves, no-added-sugar
Choice of fruit for sorbet

Chapter Eight: Quick Start Phase II VLCD Recipes

Chicken Entrees

Chicken with Orange and Fresh Basil

This delicious combination will become a favorite preparation with its intense orange flavor that's perfect with a side salad or steamed vegetable.

2 (4 oz.) chicken breast fillets
Salt and pepper to taste
Juice of 1 orange
1/2 cup low-sodium chicken broth
1/2 teaspoon orange zest
1 orange with peel, sliced into circles
2 Tablespoons basil leaves cut into julienne strips

1. Heat a nonstick skillet over medium high heat. Season the fillets with salt and pepper and lightly brown on each side without cooking through. Transfer to a plate and set aside.

2. In a small bowl combine the orange juice, broth, and zest, and pour into the skillet. Cook for 1 minute to reduce the liquid slightly. Return the chicken fillets to the skillet, top each with the orange slices and cook covered, over low heat until the chicken is cooked through and the liquid has been nearly all absorbed.

3. Transfer to a serving dish, sprinkle with the fresh basil and serve immediately.

Makes two servings

Each serving has 216 calories (1 protein, 1 fruit)

Herb Roasted Chicken with Lemon and Fennel

Delicious herbs and seasonings bring out the best in this combination that's sure to please.

1 large fennel bulb, trimmed, cored and cut into 1/4-inch thick slices
Salt and pepper to taste
2 (4 oz.) boneless chicken breasts
Juice of 1 lemon, 1 teaspoon reserved
1 large garlic clove, minced
2 teaspoons mixed dried herbs
1/2 teaspoon lemon zest

1. Preheat the oven to 375 degrees F.

2. Place the fennel slices in a single layer on the bottom of a medium baking dish and season with salt and pepper. Pour the lemon juice on top and put the chicken breasts in the middle, seasoning with salt and pepper.

3. In a small bowl combine the reserved lemon juice, garlic, herbs, and zest to form a paste and smear on top of the chicken. Cover the baking dish with a lid or foil and bake until the internal temperature of the chicken is 165 degrees F and the fennel is tender, about 35 minutes. Serve immediately.

Makes two servings

Each serving has 187 calories (1 protein, 1 vegetable)

Easy Chicken Cacciatore

Here's a zesty and delicious take on an old favorite that's sure to satisfy a taste for Italian.

2 medium tomatoes, cored, seeded and diced
2 garlic cloves, minced
1/2 teaspoon onion flakes
1 cup low-sodium chicken broth
2 teaspoons red wine vinegar
Pinch or drop of plain concentrated stevia
1/4 teaspoon each dried oregano, basil, and parsley
1 bay leaf
Salt and pepper to taste
2 (4 oz.) chicken breast fillets, each cut horizontally into 2 pieces

1. In a large nonstick skillet combine all the ingredients except for the chicken. Cook, stirring often, over medium heat until the tomatoes break down and the sauce has thickened.

2. Submerge the chicken pieces in the sauce, reduce the heat to low and cook, covered, stirring occasionally, until the chicken is cooked through and the sauce is thick. Serve immediately.

Makes two servings

Each serving has 175 calories (1 protein, 1 vegetable)

Wrapped Up Chicken Fajitas

Mexican is on the menu with these spiced up chicken fajitas wrapped in crisp lettuce leaves for a hearty and flavorful entrée.

8 oz. boneless chicken breast, cut into thin strips
Salt and pepper to taste
1/2 teaspoon chili powder
1/4 teaspoon ground cumin
1/2 cup low-sodium chicken broth
Juice of 1/2 lemon
Lettuce leaves for wrapping
Hot sauce, for seasoning (optional)

1. Heat a nonstick skillet over medium-high heat. Season the chicken pieces with salt and pepper and add to the skillet, Sprinkle with the chili powder and cumin and stir constantly to cook through, about 4 minutes.

2. Combine the broth and lemon juice and pour into the skillet stirring to coat. Remove from the heat when liquid is evaporated.

3. Serve immediately, wrapped in the lettuce leaves, with a dash of hot sauce, if desired.

Makes two servings

Each serving has 180 calories (1 protein, 1 vegetable)

VLCD Tip: Use leftover fajita chicken strips on top of salad greens for a quick lunch or dinner later in the week.

Savory Sage and Apple Chicken Burgers

Slider-size burgers are a real treat in this terrific skillet preparation that's perfect with lettuce wraps or a steamed veggie on the side.

8 oz. ground chicken breast
Salt and pepper to taste
1 teaspoon dried rubbed sage
½ teaspoon dried thyme
Dash ground cinnamon
1 medium apple, peeled and grated
1/2 cup low-sodium chicken broth

1. In a medium bowl combine the ground chicken, salt, pepper, sage, thyme, cinnamon and apple. Stir mixture well and form into 6 slider size burgers.

2. Heat a nonstick skillet over medium-high heat. Fry the burgers in the skillet, adding a little broth as needed to prevent sticking, until nicely browned on the outside and cooked through on the inside, 6 to 8 minutes in all.

3. Transfer to a plate with any accumulated juices and serve immediately.

Makes two servings

Each serving has 180 calories (1 protein, 1 fruit)

Asian Chicken Roll Ups

These easy-to-make restaurant-style roll ups are full of great flavor and a delightful kick of heat that's hard to resist.

8 oz. ground chicken breast
Salt and pepper to taste
1 large garlic clove, minced
1 teaspoon minced fresh ginger
3 Tablespoons liquid aminos
2 Tablespoons low-sodium chicken broth
Juice of 1 orange
Dash hot sauce
Whole lettuce leaves, such as butter leaf or romaine

1. Heat a nonstick skillet over medium high heat. Add the ground chicken, season with salt and pepper, and cook until no longer pink, breaking up any clumps with a fork. Add the garlic and ginger and cook a further minute.

2. In a small bowl combine the liquid aminos, broth, orange juice, and hot sauce and pour over the chicken mixture, stirring well to combine. Reduce the heat to low and cook, covered, for 10 minutes, stirring occasionally, until all liquid is absorbed. Remove from the heat.

3. To compose the roll ups mound a spoonful of the chicken mixture on lettuce leaf and and carefully fold over to eat.

Makes two servings

Each serving has 200 calories (1 protein, 1 vegetable, ½ fruit)

VLCD Tip: Try leftover Asian chicken filling as a topping for spinach salad.

Beef Entrees

Tuscan Bistecca with Lemon

Fresh rosemary and lemon make this popular steak preparation of Tuscany a real winner. Perfect when paired with garlic sautéed spinach.

Juice of 1 lemon
¼ teaspoon lemon zest
1 teaspoon finely chopped rosemary
Salt and pepper to taste
2 (4 oz.) lean steaks such as sirloin or tenderloin

1. In a shallow dish combine the lemon juice, zest, and rosemary. Season the steak with salt and pepper and rub with the lemon mixture. Set aside for 30 minutes, turning over halfway through.

2. Prepare a grill or broiler. Cook the steak to desired doneness (about 5 minutes per side for medium-rare). Remove from grill and let rest for 4 minutes before serving.

Makes two servings

Each serving has 220 calories (1 protein)

VLCD Tip: Make a hearty beef salad later in the week with your second steak.

Chinese Orange Beef Stir Fry

Fast and easy to make, this tasty beef dish gets a double dose of orange flavor from both the juice and the zest, as well as a delightful zing from red pepper flakes.

8 oz. lean beef steak, such as tenderloin, sliced thin
Salt and pepper to taste
1 tcaspoon onion flakes
4 cups thinly sliced Napa (Chinese) cabbage
1/2 cup low-sodium beef broth
3 Tablespoons liquid aminos
Juice of 1 orange
1 teaspoon orange zest
Dash red pepper flakes
Segments from 1 orange, for garnish

1. Heat a nonstick skillet over medium-high heat. Season the beef with salt, pepper, and onion flakes, add to the skillet, and cook, stirring often, until slightly browned but not cooked through. Transfer to a clean plate.

2. Add the cabbage to the skillet, season with salt and pepper, and cook, stirring, for 3 minutes.

3. Combine the remaining ingredients except the orange segments in a small bowl and pour into the skillet with the cabbage. Return the beef to the skillet, stir well, reduce heat to low, cover and cook until vegetables are crisp tender and beef is cooked to desired doneness, about 3 minutes.

4. Taste for the addition of salt and pepper, transfer to a serving dish, and garnish with the orange segments.

Makes two servings

Each serving has 254 calories (1 protein, 1 vegetable, 1 fruit)

Skewered Steak and Red Onions

A quick marinade and grilling brings out the fabulous flavor of this kebab-style entrée that's both satisfying and delicious.

8 oz. lean beef, such as tenderloin, cubed
2 medium red onion, peeled and cut into chunks
1/3 cup red wine vinegar
1 Tablespoon liquid aminos
1/8 teaspoon plain concentrated stevia
¼ teaspoon garlic powder
1/2 teaspoon dried oregano
1 teaspoon bottled horseradish
Salt and pepper to taste

1. Place the cubed beef and onion chunks in a shallow dish. In a small bowl whisk together the vinegar, liquid aminos, stevia, garlic powder, oregano, horseradish, salt and pepper, and pour over the beef and onions. Marinate for 30 minutes, stirring occasionally.

2. Preheat a grlll or broiler. Thread the beef and onions on a metal skewer and pat dry. Grill kebabs to desired doneness (about 4 minutes per side for rare), turning the skewers occasionally to cook evenly. Serve immediately.

Makes two servings

Each serving has 235 calories (1 protein, 1 vegetable)

Super Beef Chili

Enjoy a traditional, flavorful bowl of chili with this fabulous VLCD version that's easy to make and even easier to eat.

8 oz. lean (95%) ground beef
1/2 teaspoon onion flakes
1/2 teaspoon garlic granules
1 Tablespoon chili powder
1 teaspoon paprika
1/4 teaspoon ground cumin
Dash cayenne pepper
Pinch of salt
1 cup low sodium beef broth
2 medium tomatoes, cored, seeded, and diced
Pinch or drop of plain concentrated stevia

1. In a large nonstick skillet over medium-high heat, brown the ground beef, using a fork to break up any clumps. Add the onion flakes, garlic granules, chili powder, paprika, cumin, cayenne, and salt, stir well to combine, and cook a further minute.

2. In a medium bowl combine the broth, tomatoes, and stevia and pour the mixture into the skillet, stirring well to combine.

3. Cook over low heat, stirring often, until the liquid is mostly absorbed and the beef is flavorful, about 20 minutes. Taste for seasoning and serve immediately.

Makes two servings

Each serving has 194 calories (1 protein, 1 vegetable)

The Big Bodacious Burger

This amazing burger that's loaded with bursts of flavor is even tastier when served alongside Tangy Apple Slaw.

For the Burger:
  4 oz. lean (95%) ground beef
  Salt and pepper to taste
  1/2 teaspoon each onion flakes and garlic granules
  1/4 teaspoon dried mustard
  1/4 teaspoon dried thyme
  Dash cayenne pepper

For Deglazing:
  1 Tablespoon red wine vinegar
  1 Tablespoon low sodium-beef broth or water
  2 teaspoons liquid aminos

1. In a medium bowl combine all the burger ingredients mixing well with your hands. Shape into a burger and set aside.

2. Heat a nonstick skillet on high and brown the burger on both sides. Reduce the heat to low, cover, and cook to desired doneness (about 4 minutes per side for medium-well).

3. In a small bowl combine the vinegar, broth, and liquid aminos. Remove the lid from the skillet and sprinkle the vinegar mixture over the burger and continue to cook as the liquid is absorbed, about 1 minute more. Transfer to a plate and serve immediately.

Makes one serving

Each serving has 158 calories (1 protein)

Seafood Entrees

Tilapia with Strawberry Salsa

This unusual combination that's also fast and easy will become a favorite entrée in no time. Perfect when served with a side of steamed asparagus or a green salad.

  8 oz. tilapia fillet or other firm white fleshed fish
  Salt and pepper to taste

Salsa for one serving:
  1 Tablespoon finely chopped fresh mint
  Juice of half a lemon
  2 Tablespoons red wine vinegar
  1/8 teaspoon plain concentrated stevia
  10 medium strawberries, stemmed and diced

1. Preheat an oven broiler to high. Line a baking sheet with foil and place fish in middle. Season with salt and pepper.

2. In a small bowl combine the chopped mint, lemon juice, and vinegar, and stevia drops. Add the strawberries, toss to coat and set aside.

3. Broil the fish until cooked and just flaking, about 5 minutes.

4. Transfer to a plate, spoon the strawberry salsa over, and serve immediately.

Makes two servings

Each serving has 160 calories (1 protein, 1 fruit)

VLCD Tip: If grilling fish ahead for a meal later in the week, make extra salsa fresh that night.

Broiled Lemon Garlic Shrimp

Reminiscent of shrimp scampi, you'll love the intense garlic flavor and fresh lemon taste.

8 oz. large shrimp, shelled and deveined
Salt and pepper to taste
2 large garlic cloves, peeled and minced
Juice of 1 lemon
2 teaspoons white wine vinegar
1 teaspoon chopped fresh parsley

1. Preheat the oven broiler to high.

2. Line a small rimmed baking sheet with foil. Place the shrimp on the foil in a single layer and season with salt and pepper.

3. In a small bowl stir together the garlic, lemon juice, vinegar, and chopped parsley. Spoon or brush evenly over the shrimp.

4. Broil until the shrimp are pink, turning the sheet pan to cook evenly, 3 to 5 minutes.

5. Transfer to a dish and serve immediately.

Makes two servings

Each serving has 120 calories (1 protein)

VLCD Tip: Feature your leftover shrimp as a salad topping for spinach or mixed lettuce.

Orange Soy Glazed Shrimp

Sweet orange is just the ticket for this super flavorful skewered shrimp dish that's sure to satisfy.

For the Glaze:
   Juice of 2 oranges
   1/2 cup liquid aminos
   2 medium garlic cloves, minced
   1 Tablespoon finely chopped fresh ginger
   ½ teaspoon orange zest
   Dash red pepper flakes (optional)
   8 oz. large shrimp, shelled and deveined
   Salt and pepper to taste

1. Make the glaze by combining all the glaze ingredients in a small saucepan and simmering until slightly reduced and thickened, about 5 minutes. Set aside.

2. Thread the shrimp on metal skewers and season with salt and pepper. Prepare an indoor or outdoor grill with a nonstick rack.

3. Grill the shrimp, while brushing frequently with the glaze, until pink, about 2 minutes per side. Transfer skewers to a serving plate. Boil remaining glaze for 1 minute and pour over cooked shrimp. Serve immediately.

   Makes two servings

   Each serving has 227 calories (1 protein, 1 fruit)

Petit Baked Crab Cakes

These scrumptious two-bite crab delights are great for making in batches ahead of time for freezing and reheating.

8 oz. lump crab meat, picked over for cartilage and shells
1/2 teaspoon Old Bay Seasoning
Pinch of salt
2 teaspoons dried mixed herbs
Juice of 1/2 lemon
2 Tablespoons milk
2 breadsticks, crushed into fine crumbs

1. Preheat the oven to 350 degrees F.

2. In a medium bowl combine the crab, Old Bay, salt, herbs and lemon juice and stir gently. Add the milk and breadstick crumbs and lightly stir in.

3. Form small balls and place in a mini muffin tin, gently flattening the tops. Bake until golden and hot, 15 to 20 minutes. Carefully remove from the tin and serve immediately, or cool and freeze in an airtight container.

Makes two servings

Each serving has 158 calories (1 protein)

Vegetarian Entrees

Tomato Bruschetta Omelet

The fresh flavors of tomato, garlic, and basil highlight this wonderful omelet recipe. Try filling with garlic sautéed spinach or chard on other occasions.

For the Tomato Bruschetta:
    1 medium tomato, cored, seeded and diced
    1 garlic clove, minced
    Salt and pepper to taste
    2 teaspoons red wine vinegar
    Pinch dried oregano
    2 teaspoons chopped fresh basil leaves
    1 whole egg plus 3 egg whites

1.   In a small bowl combine all the Bruschetta ingredients and stir well. Set aside.

2. In a medium bowl, whisk together the egg and egg whites and a pinch of salt and pepper. Heat a nonstick skillet over medium heat. Pour the egg mixture into the skillet and turn the heat to low.

3. Cook the egg evenly by lifting the firm edges to allow the wet egg mixture to reach the bottom of the pan. Cover and continue to cook over the very lowest of heat until the top surface has set.

4. Spoon the Bruschetta mixture onto one side of the omelet and carefully flip the other side over with a spatula. Cover and cook a further minute. Slide onto a plate and serve immediately.

Makes one serving

Each servings has 155 calories (1 protein, 1 vegetable)

Easy Onion Frittata

This frittata requires no flipping, making it simple and quick to prepare.

2 cups sliced onions
Salt and pepper to taste
1 teaspoon dried thyme
Juice of 1 orange
2 whole eggs plus 6 egg whites
1 orange, unpeeled, cut into circles

1. Heat a nonstick skillet over medium-high heat. Add the onions, salt, pepper, and thyme, and cook, stirring often, until the onions have softened, about 6 minutes. Add a little water if necessary to prevent sticking.

2. Pour the orange juice over the onion mixture and cook a further minute. In a medium bowl whisk together the eggs and egg whites with a pinch of salt and pepper. Pour into the skillet and move the onions evenly around.

3. Reduce the heat to low, cover, and cook until the bottom is lightly browned and the top is nearly set, 5 to 8 minutes. Remove the lid and place the skillet under a low broiler for a brief few seconds to finish cooking the top.

4. Loosen the sides of the frittata with a spatula and slide onto a plate. Serve immediately with the orange slices as garnish.

Makes two servings

Each serving has 215 calories (1 protein, 1 vegetable, 1 fruit)

Sweet Strawberry Souffle Omelet

You'll feel as if you're eating dessert for dinner with this wonderfully satisfying omelet full of juicy strawberries.

10 strawberries, stemmed and diced
1 Tablespoon water
1/8 teaspoon concentrated stevia
1 whole egg
3 egg whites
Pinch of salt

1. In a medium bowl stir together the strawberries, water, and stevia. Set aside for 15 minutes.

2. In a large bowl whisk the whole egg until pale yellow. In another large bowl beat the egg whites with the salt using an electric beater to soft peaks. Fold the beaten egg whites in batches, into the beaten egg until well combined but still large in volume.

3. Heat a nonstick skillet over medium heat. Pour the egg mixture into the skillet, spread out evenly, reduce the heat to low, cover and cook until set, 4 to 6 minutes.

4. Spoon the strawberry mixture over the omelet and fold over. Slide out of the skillet onto a plate and serve immediately.

Makes one serving

Each serving has 170 calories (1 protein, 1 fruit)

Apple Cottage Cheese Dip

For those who prefer to "dip" into their protein, this wonderful treat is perfect for a light lunch or supper.

For the Dip:
    ½ apple, peeled and grated
    1 teaspoon lemon juice
    1/8 teaspoon concentrated stevia
    ½ nonfat cottage cheese
    Dash ground cinnamon

For Dipping:

    ½ apple, cored and sliced
    Celery sticks (about 2 cups)
    Melba toast (optional)

1. In a small bowl combine the grated apple, lemon juice, and stevia. Set aside for 10 minutes.

2. Stir the cottage cheese into the apple mixture and transfer to a small dipping bowl. Top with a dash of cinnamon and refrigerate until ready to serve.

3. Meanwhile prepare a plate with the sliced apple, celery sticks, and Melba, if using. Place the bowl with the dip in the middle and serve immediately.

Makes one serving

Each serving has 222 calories (1 protein, 1 vegetable, 1 fruit)

So-y Delicious Chili

Plain soy patties take on the zesty flavors of Mexico in this easy chili dish that's both satisfying and delicious.

2 medium tomatoes, cored, seeded and diced
1 garlic clove, minced
½ teaspoon onion flakes
1 Tablespoon chili powder
1 teaspoon paprika
¼ teaspoon ground cumin
Salt and pepper to taste
1 cup low-sodium vegetable broth
2 (4 oz.) soy patties, cooked and crumbled

1. In a medium saucepan combine the tomatoes, garlic, and onion flakes and bring to a simmer. Cook over low heat, stirring often, until the tomatoes begin to break down, about 4 minutes. Add the chili powder, paprika, cumin, salt, and pepper, and cook a further minute.

2. Add the broth to the tomato mixture and bring to a simmer. Stir in the soy patties and cook over low heat, stirring occasionally, until thickened, about 20 minutes. Taste for seasoning and serve immediately.

Makes two servings

Each serving has 133 calories (1 protein, 1 vegetable)

Spinach Soy Patties with Lemon Sauce Glaze

Doctored-up soy patties get a boost of flavor from garlic sautéed spinach and a tangy lemon glaze.

3 cups baby spinach leaves
1 garlic clove, minced
Salt and pepper to taste
2 (4 oz.) soy patties, defrosted (if necessary) and crumbled
¼ teaspoon lemon zest
½ cup low-sodium vegetable broth
Juice of ½ lemon
1/8 teaspoon concentrated stevia
½ lemon with rind, sliced thin

1. In a large nonstick skillet over medium heat, sauté the spinach with the garlic and salt and pepper until just wilted. Set aside to cool.

2. Chop the spinach mixture and combine in a medium bowl with the soy patties and lemon zest. Form into 4 patties and refrigerate for 20 minutes.

3. Heat a nonstick skillet over medium-high heat and fry the patties, browning on both sides, about 5 minutes in all. Combine the broth, lemon juice, and stevia in a small bowl and add to the skillet, swirling to coat the patties. Place the lemon slices on top of the patties, cover, reduce the heat to low, and cook a further 2 minutes. Serve immediately.

Makes two servings

Each serving has 125 calories (1 protein, ½ vegetable)

Sides and Salads

Cream of Fennel Soup

Here fennel, the anise-flavored vegetable, teams up with sweet orange and piquant coriander for a super result.

3 cups low-sodium chicken or vegetable broth
1 cup water
2 medium oranges, peeled, seeded, and roughly chopped
¼ teaspoon ground coriander
3 cups roughly chopped fennel, tough stalks removed
Salt and pepper to taste
Fennel fronds for garnish

1. Combine the broth, water, oranges, and coriander in a soup pot and bring to a boil over high heat.

2. Stir in the fennel, reduce the heat to low, cover and cook until the fennel is fork tender, 20 to 25 minutes.

3. Transfer the mixture to a blender, working in batches if necessary, and puree until completely smooth.

4. Return to a clean saucepan, season to taste with salt and pepper, and serve immediately, garnished with fennel fronds.

Makes two servings

Each serving has 120 calories (1 vegetable, 1 fruit)

French Onion Soup

Diced apple and stevia add a hint of sweetness, while fresh thyme compliments the flavors of this old favorite.

2 medium onions, peeled, halved, and thinly sliced
Salt and pepper to taste
1 medium apple, peeled, cored and cut into small dice
1 sprig fresh thyme
1 garlic clove, minced
2 Tablespoons apple cider vinegar
1/8 teaspoon concentrated stevia
4 cups low-sodium beef or vegetable broth
1 teaspoon chopped parsley leaves (optional)

1. Heat a large nonstick skillet over medium-high heat. Add the onions, season with salt and pepper, and cook, stirring often, until soft and lightly browned, about 30 minutes. Reduce heat as necessary to prevent burning.

2. Add the apple and thyme, stir to combine, and continue to cook for 3 to 5 minutes. Add the garlic and cook a further minute.

3. In a small bowl combine the vinegar and Stevia and pour this into the skillet, stirring constantly. Transfer to a saucepan and add the broth to the onion mixture. Bring to simmer and allow to cook, over low heat for 10 minutes, stirring occasionally.

4. Season to taste with salt and pepper and serve immediately, topped with a pinch of chopped parsley, if using.

Makes two servings

Each serving has 120 calories (1 vegetable, ½ fruit)

Tangy Apple Slaw

Sweet and tangy with the fresh crunch of apple and cabbage, this cole slaw gets better the longer it sits.

4 cups thinly shredded cabbage
2 apples, cored and cut into small dice
1/2 cup apple cider vinegar
2 Tablespoons lemon juice
¼ teaspoon concentrated stevia
Salt and pepper to taste
1/4 teaspoon poppy seeds (optional)

1. Combine the cabbage and apple in a medium bowl.

2. In a small bowl, whisk together the vinegar, lemon juice, and stevia. Pour over the cabbage mixture, season to taste with salt and pepper, add the poppy seeds if using, and stir gently to coat.

3. Refrigerate at least 1 hour, occasionally tossing, before serving.

Makes two servings

Each serving has 134 calories (1 vegetable, 1 fruit)

Minty Radish and Grapefruit Slaw

This delicious combination benefits from a touch of cool mint and sweet stevia for a slaw that's simply perfect with any grilled entree.

2 cups red radishes, trimmed, and diced small
1/2 grapefruit, peeled, seeded, and chopped, juice reserved
Juice of 1/2 lemon
1/8 teaspoon concentrated stevia
Salt to taste
1 teaspoon chopped fresh mint leaves

1. Combine the radishes and grapefruit in a mixing bowl. In a small bowl whisk together the reserved grapefruit juice, lemon juice, and stevia.

2. Pour the dressing over the radish mixture, season with salt, and toss well to coat. Allow to refrigerate for 30 minutes before serving, topped with the chopped mint.

Makes one serving

Each serving has 145 calories (1 vegetable, 1 fruit)

Cucumber and Orange Salad

Crisp and refreshing, this quick salad makes a great accompaniment for grilled chicken or steak.

1 large cucumber, peeled and sliced thin (about 2 cups)
1 orange, peeled and segmented
1/4 cup white wine vinegar
1/4 teaspoon concentrated stevia
Salt and pepper to taste
1 teaspoon finely chopped fresh parsley

1. Combine the cucumber and orange segments in a medium bowl.

2. In a small bowl, whisk together the vinegar and stevia. Pour over the cucumber mixture, season with salt and pepper, add the parsley, and toss gently.

3. Refrigerate for 30 minutes before serving.

Makes one serving

Each serving has 115 calories (1 vegetable, 1 fruit)

Chapter Nine: Quick Start Phase III Maintenance Recipes

Poultry Entrees

Super Juicy Roast Lemon Chicken

Tangy lemon and flavorful onion help to seal in moistness in this delicious rosemary-scented entrée featuring roasted chicken leg quarters.

2 lemons, cut into 1/4-inch slices
4 rosemary sprigs
1 small onion, thinly sliced
4 chicken leg quarters
1 Tablespoon olive oil
Salt and pepper to taste

1. Preheat the oven to 400 dg F.

2. Place the lemon slices in a single layer in the bottom of a roasting pan. Top with the rosemary springs.

3. Tuck the onion slices under the skin of each chicken quarter. Rub each quarter with olive oil and season with salt and pepper.

4. Place each quarter on top of the lemons and rosemary. Roast in the oven until the skin is golden and an internal read thermometer registers 175 dg F in the thighs, 40 to 50 minutes, basting occasionally with the accumulated pan juices.

5. Remove from the oven and allow to rest for 10 minutes before serving. Remove skin before eating, if desired. Top with the lemon slices.

Makes four servings, 367 calories each

Moroccan Chicken Breasts

Exotically spiced and deliciously accompanied by roasted dried plums, this Middle Eastern dish will quickly become a dinner favorite.

1 Tablespoon olive oil
1/2 teaspoon ground cumin
1/2 teaspoon ground cinnamon
1/4 teaspoon ground cardamom
Salt and pepper to taste
2 split chicken breasts, skin removed
8 dried plums (prunes)
Juice of 1 orange
1 Tablespoon balsamic vinegar

1. Preheat the oven to 425 degrees F.

2. In a small bowl whisk together olive oil, cumin, cinnamon, and cardamom. Season the chicken with salt and pepper and place breast side up in a medium roasting pan. Drizzle oil mixture over top and roast chicken for 15 minutes.

3. Meanwhile, combine the prunes, orange juice and balsamic vinegar in a bowl and soak for at least 10 minutes. After the chicken has roasted for 15 minutes, add the prune mixture to the roasting pan, stir, and continue to cook, occasionally basting with the prune mixture, until the chicken reaches an internal temperature of 165 degrees F, or is golden and firm to the touch, about 20 minutes more.

4. Remove from the oven and allow to rest for 10 minutes before serving.

Makes two servings, 440 calories each

Quick and Easy Chicken Stew

This hearty stew will warm your insides and satisfy a hungry appetite for comfort food in no time.

2 Tablespoons olive oil
1 medium onion, diced
1 large celery stalk, diced
1 large carrot, diced
4 garlic cloves, chopped
1 1/2 cups no-salt-added diced tomatoes with juice
1 cup low-sodium chicken broth
1/2 cup water
¼ teaspoon ground turmeric
Pinch sugar substitute
1 lb boneless, skinless chicken breasts, cut into bite-size pieces
Salt and pepper to taste
1 Tablespoon chopped fresh parsley

1. Heat oil in a large heavy-bottomed pot over medium heat. Add onion, celery, and carrots and cook, stirring occasionally, until softened, about 6 minutes. Add garlic and cook a further minute.

2. Stir in tomatoes, broth, water, turmeric and sweetener. Increase heat to high and bring to a boil. Reduce heat to medium-low and simmer, stirring occasionally, for 5 minutes.

3. Add chicken and simmer, covered, until vegetables and chicken are just cooked through and stew is piping hot, about 12 minutes. Season with salt and pepper, and serve sprinkled with parsley.

Makes four servings, 253 calories each

Terrific Turkey Loaf

Deliciously moist with a hint of sage and the sweet taste of sautéed onion, this tasty turkey loaf is healthy and satisfying.

1 Tablespoon olive oil
1 medium onion, finely chopped
Salt and pepper to taste
2 teaspoons rubbed sage leaves
1 teaspoon dried thyme
1 lb. ground turkey
1 large egg white, beaten
2 teaspoons prepared mustard
Dash ground paprika
2 Tablespoons ground flaxseed
1/4 cup chicken broth
1 Tablespoon Worcestershire sauce

1. Preheat the oven to 325 dg F.

2. Heat the olive oil in a skillet over medium heat. Add the onion, season with salt and pepper, and cook until soft, about 2 minutes. Add the sage and thyme and cook a further minute. Set aside to cool.

3. In a medium mixing bowl combine the ground turkey, egg white, mustard, paprika and ground flaxseeds, stirring well to combine. In a small bowl combine the broth and Worcestershire and add to the loaf mixture. Add the onion mixture and stir well.

4. Transfer to a glass or ceramic 8 x 3-inch loaf pan and pat down to remove any air pockets. Cover with foil and bake until an instant read thermometer inserted in the middle reaches 165 dg F, 45 to 55 minutes. Remove from the oven and allow to rest for 10 minutes before slicing and serving.

Makes four servings, 240 calories each

Phase III Maintenance Recipes

Meat Entrees

Teriyaki Beef with Snow Peas

Thin slices of beef take on abundant flavor when marinated before cooking in this easy stir-fry recipe full of delicious and healthy Asian vegetables.

8 oz beef tenderloin or sirloin, sliced into thin strips
1 Tablespoon olive oil
1 bunch scallions, ends trimmed and cut into 1 1/2-inch lengths
1/2 cup shredded carrots
Salt and pepper to taste
1 cup fresh snow peas
1/4 teaspoon sesame seeds
For the Marinade:
1/2 cup low-sodium soy sauce or liquid aminos
1 Tablespoon plain rice vinegar
1/8 teaspoon sugar substitute
2 teaspoons minced fresh ginger
1 large garlic clove, minced

1. In a medium glass baking dish, combine the marinade ingredients and stir well with a fork. Add the beef slices and allow to marinate for at least 30 minutes, turning them over halfway through.

2. Heat the oil in a wok or large nonstick skillet over high heat. Remove the beef from the marinade and lightly pat dry with a paper towel. Fry it in the oil (do not stir-fry or move around in the pan) until the edges are golden and crisp, about 3 minutes per side. Transfer to the middle of a large heated platter.

3. Add a touch more oil to the wok or skillet and heat to nearly smoking. Add the scallions and carrots, sprinkle with salt and pepper, and stir-fry over high heat for 2 minutes. Add the snow peas, season again with salt and pepper, and continue to stir-fry another minute. Add the sesame seeds and transfer the vegetables to the outside of the platter, surrounding the beef, and serve immediately.

Makes two servings, 351 calories each

Hearty Beef Stroganoff

A delicious and creamy sauce engulfs tender strips of steak in this wonderful version of an old favorite.

1 Tablespoon olive oil
1 lb. beef round steak, trimmed and cut into 1/2-inch strips
Salt and pepper to taste
1 medium onion, diced
1 package (10 oz) white mushrooms, wiped clean, stemmed, and halved
1 cup tomato sauce
1 cup low-sodium beef broth
1/3 cup plain reduced-fat Greek yogurt

1. Heat the oil in a large non-stick skillet over medium-high heat. Add the beef, season with salt and pepper, and cook, stirring occasionally, until lightly browned, about 5 minutes. Remove beef with a slotted spoon and set aside.

2. Add the onion to the skillet and cook, stirring often, until softened, about 3 minutes. Add the mushrooms to the skillet and cook 2 minutes more.

3. Stir in the tomato sauce and broth, bring to a boil. Add the browned beef, and reduce the heat to low. Cook, covered, until beef is fork tender, about 1 hour. Occasionally stir to prevent sticking and add a little water if necessary.

4. Use a slotted spoon to transfer the meat and mushrooms to a warm serving bowl. Add the yogurt to the skillet and whisk to combine. Allow to simmer and thicken for 2 minutes. Taste the sauce for seasoning and pour over the beef and mushrooms. Serve immediately.

Makes four servings, 260 calories each

Tangy Stuffed Peppers

*This time-honored entrée in a tangy tomato sauce gets a
touch of sweetness from a surprising source.*

2 large green bell peppers, halved, cored and seeded
2 teaspoons olive oil
1lb. ground beef or veal
1 small onion, minced
1/4 cup grated carrot
1 small celery stalk, finely chopped
Salt and pepper to taste
1 garlic clove, minced
1 teaspoon dried parsley
Dash ground allspice
1 1/2 cups tomato sauce
1/4 cup low sodium beef broth
2 Tablespoons dried cranberries
Dash paprika

1. Bring a medium pot of water to the boil. Drop in the
bell pepper halves and cook for 2 minutes, then remove
with a slotted spoon and place on paper towels to dry.
Place cut side up in a 9 x 13-inch casserole. Preheat the
oven to 350 degrees F.

2. Heat the olive oil in a medium nonstick skillet over
medium-high heat and add the beef or veal, onion,
carrot, celery, salt, and pepper. Using a fork, break up
the meat into fine pieces as it cooks.

3. When the meat is lightly browned, stir in the garlic
and cook a further minute. Remove from the heat and
stir in the parsley, allspice, and 1/4 cup of the tomato
sauce. Spoon the mixture into the bell pepper halves,
pressing firmly into mounds.

4. Pour the remaining tomato sauce into the empty
skillet and stir in the broth, cranberries, and paprika.
Cook over low heat until just bubbly and pour evenly
over the stuffed peppers. Cover the casserole with foil,
and bake until the peppers are fork tender and the
stuffing is piping hot, about 40 minutes. Serve
immediately.

Makes four servings, 282 calories each

Phase III Maintenance Recipes

Pork Chops with Apples and Kraut

This terrific dish with chunky sweet apples is a snap to make and super delectable to eat as well.

2 Tablespoons olive oil
8 thin cut loin or rib pork chops (1 lb. total), trimmed of fat
Salt and pepper to taste
2 large Red or Golden Delicious apples, cored and cut into eighths
Dash of cinnamon
One 15 oz. can sauerkraut, drained

1. Preheat the oven to 375 dg F.

2. Heat the oil in a nonstick skillet over medium-high heat. Season pork chops with salt and pepper and fry in skillet until lightly browned, about 2 minutes per side. Transfer to a 9 x 13-inch casserole.

3. Add apples to skillet, sprinkle with cinnamon, and cook, scraping up browned bits, for 2 minutes just until they begin to color. Transfer to the edges of the casserole.

4. Add sauerkraut to skillet and cook, stirring, until heated through, about 3 minutes. Remove from the heat and place sauerkraut on top of the pork chops in the casserole to cover.

5. Bake until pork chops are no longer pink and apples are brown and fork tender, about 35 minutes. Serve immediately.

Makes four servings, 330 calories each

Seafood Entrees

Lemon-Lime Fish Fillet with Salsa

Prepared salsa makes this dish a real snap while the tang of citrus wakes up the terrific Mexican spices.

One 8 oz. scrod or cod fillet, cut into 2 pieces
Juice of ½ lime
Juice of ½ lemon
Dash each ground cumin and chili powder
Salt and pepper to taste
1/2 cup purchased tomato salsa
1 tablespoon chopped fresh cilantro leaves

1. Preheat the broiler and position the oven rack 4 to 5 inches below the flame.

2. On an aluminum foil-lined baking sheet that has been lightly coated with cooking spray or oil, place the fish in a single layer. Combine the lime and lemon juice and drizzle over the fish. Sprinkle with the cumin and chili powder, and season with salt and pepper.

3. Broil, shifting the pan a few times to cook evenly, until the fish is firm to the touch and golden brown around the edges, 5 to 6 minutes.

4. Remove from the broiler, transfer to warm serving plates, and spoon the salsa evenly over the fish, garnishing with the cilantro. Serve immediately.

Makes two servings, 115 calories each

Seared Ahi Tuna with Wasabi Dressing

Fans of sashimi will adore this easy preparation for tuna made with the zing of wasabi and the zest of orange.

2 teaspoons wasabi powder, more or less to taste
1 Tablespoon hot water
2 Tablespoons low-sodium soy sauce or liquid aminos
Juice of 1/2 an orange
1 Tablespoon olive oil
Two 4 oz. ahi or sushi-grade tuna fillets
Pinch sea salt and pepper to taste
2 cups watercress to serve
½ teaspoon sesame seeds

1. In a small bowl whisk together wasabi and water until smooth. Whisk in soy sauce and orange juice and set aside.

2. Lightly coat tuna fillets with some of the oil, season with salt and pepper, and set aside.

3. Brush remaining oil in a nonstick skillet. Over high heat, cook tuna until crust is browned but fish is still pink inside, 2 to 3 minutes per side. Transfer to a cutting board.

4. To serve, scatter watercress over 2 plates, slice tuna and place on top, then drizzle wasabi dressing over all and sprinkle with the sesame seeds.

Makes two servings, 203 calories each

Sensational Salmon Burger

This healthy and delicious alternative to the classic burger is perfect for the grill or broiler.

8 oz. boneless, skinless, salmon fillet, cut into large cubes
Salt and pepper to taste
1 large egg white, slightly beaten
1 Tablespoon lemon juice
1/4 teaspoon Old Bay Seasoning
2 teaspoons each chopped fresh dill and cilantro

1.   Place all the ingredients in a food processor and using the pulse button, chop until just combined. Transfer to a cutting board or clean plate. Mold the salmon mixture into the shape of 2 burgers, place on waxed paper, and set in the fridge for 10 to 15 minutes.

2. Heat a grill or broiler to medium-high. Lightly coat the grates or the bottom of a broiler pan with oil. Grill or broil the burgers until they are firm to the touch and lightly golden, 3 to 4 minutes per side. Serve immediately.

Makes two servings, 214 calories each

Super Shrimp Gumbo

Full of spicy tomato flavor, this gumbo couldn't be easier to prepare. Cool things off with a dollop of creamy nonfat Greek yogurt on top, if desired.

1 lb medium shrimp, shelled and deveined
1 teaspoon Creole seasoning blend
1 Tablespoon olive oil
1 small onion, diced
1 small green bell pepper, diced
1 medium celery stalk, trimmed and diced
Salt and pepper to taste
1 garlic clove, minced
1 can (15 oz) crushed tomatoes
1/2 cup water
Pinch sugar substitute
1 Tablespoon tomato paste
1/2 teaspoon dried oregano

1. Place shrimp in a large bowl and sprinkle with the creole seasoning. Set aside.

2. Heat the oil in a heavy-bottomed pot over medium-high heat. Add the onion, green pepper, and celery, season with salt and pepper, and cook over medium heat until the vegetables are softened, stirring often, about 4 minutes. Add the garlic and cook, stirring, a further minute.

3. Stir in the tomatoes, water, sweetener, tomato paste, and oregano and bring to a boil. Reduce heat to medium-low and simmer for 15 minutes, stirring occasionally.

4. Add the shrimp, stir well, and simmer until just cooked, 3 to 4 minutes. Remove the shrimp with a slotted spoon and transfer to a warm serving bowl.

5. Continue to simmer the sauce until well thickened, about 5 minutes more. Taste for seasoning, pour over the cooked shrimp and serve immediately.

Makes four servings, 173 calories each

Phase III Maintenance Recipes

Vegetarian Entrees

Eggplant Rollatini

This hearty vegetarian Italian dish is baked and not fried for a lower fat and cleaner tasting result that you'll absolutely love.

1 large eggplant
2 Tablespoons olive oil
Salt and pepper to taste
1 cup large curd cottage cheese
1 teaspoon chopped parsley
1 large egg, slightly beaten
1 1/2 cups no-added-sugar marinara sauce

1. Preheat the oven to 350 degrees F. Lightly brush a large baking sheet with some of the oil and set aside.

2. Cut the ends off the eggplant and peel. Slicing downwards, cut into 1/4-inch thick slices to make 4 to 6 complete slices (discard end pieces or reserve for another recipe). Place the eggplant on the oiled sheet and brush with more of the oil. Sprinkle with salt and pepper, and bake until fork tender and lightly browned around the edges, turning halfway through and brushing more oil as needed, about 25 minutes. Set aside to cool.

3. In a medium bowl combine the cottage cheese, parsley, and egg, and season with salt and pepper. Lay the cooked eggplant slices on a flat surface and distribute the cheese filling among the slices by placing a dollop in the middle of each. Beginning at the short end of the slice, roll up the eggplant carefully but firmly to enclose the filling.

4. Spoon half the marinara sauce in the bottom of a medium casserole and place the roll ups, seam side down, in the dish next to each other, but not touching. Pour the remaining sauce over all, and bake until the sauce is bubbly and the filling is hot, about 20 minutes. Serve immediately.

Makes two servings, 374 calories each

Indonesian Vegetarian Stew

Exotic flavors highlight this medley of nutritious vegetables and tofu that has a good amount of heat for spicy food lovers.

1 Tablespoon olive oil
1/2 medium onion, chopped
1/2 medium red bell pepper, cored, seeded, and diced
Salt and pepper to taste
1 Tablespoon minced fresh ginger
2 garlic cloves, minced
1/2 small jalapeno pepper, seeded and minced
1 Tablespoon curry powder
1/2 teaspoon ground turmeric
1/4 teaspoon coriander
2 cups vegetable broth
1/2 cup unsweetened coconut milk
1/8 teaspoon sugar substitute
8 drops plain Stevia
1/2 cup sliced carrots
1/2 cup cauliflower florets
8 oz. extra-firm tofu, drained, cut into small cubes

1. Heat the oil in a large pot over medium-high heat. Add the onion, bell pepper, salt and pepper, and cook, stirring often, until softened, about 3 minutes.

2. Add the ginger, garlic, and jalapeno, and cook, stirring, a further minute. Add the curry powder, turmeric, and coriander, and stir well to coat the vegetables.

3. Stir in the broth, coconut milk, and sweetener, and bring to a low boil. Add the carrots and cauliflower, reduce the heat to low, cover, and simmer until the vegetables are tender, about 10 minutes. Gently stir in the tofu and simmer a further 2 minutes.

4. Remove vegetables and tofu with a slotted spoon and transfer to a serving bowl. Taste the sauce for seasoning and adjust if necessary. If necessary, simmer to reduce sauce slightly, then pour over the vegetable mixture and serve.

Makes two servings, 457 calories each

Phase III Maintenance Recipes

Crustless Quiche with Sun Dried Tomatoes

No crust – no problem – in this great tasting dish that's easy to vary and always meatless for vegetarian eaters.

1 teaspoon olive oil
1/2 cup whipped cottage cheese
4 large eggs
2/3 cup milk or unsweetened plain soymilk
Salt and pepper to taste
Dash of nutmeg
1/2 teaspoon Herbs de Provence
1/4 cup sun-dried tomatoes (not marinated) minced

1. Preheat the oven to 350 degrees F. Lightly coat an 8 or 9-inch round cake pan with the oil.

2. In a medium bowl whisk together the remaining ingredients and pour into the prepared cake pan. Bake until the quiche is set and lightly browned on top, 25 to 30 minutes. Cut into quarters and serve.

Makes four servings, 125 calories each

Herbed Portobello Burger

Mushroom lovers adore the "meatiness" of a Portobello mushroom cap and here it fills in nicely for the standard beef burger, flavored with bold and aromatic herbs.

1 large Portobello mushroom cap, stem removed
1 Tablespoon olive oil
1 teaspoon tarragon vinegar
1 teaspoon dried mixed herbs
Salt and pepper to taste
To serve:
Sugar-free ketchup or dressing
Lettuce leaves and sliced tomato

1. Using a teaspoon, carefully scrape away the dark gills under the mushroom cap. In a small bowl stir together the remaining ingredients.

2. Prepare an outdoor or indoor grill to medium-high. Grill the mushroom cap, brushing with the oil mixture, until fork tender, about 5 minutes. Transfer to a serving dish and serve as desired.

Makes one serving, 154 calories each

Sides and Salads

Creamy Broccoli Soup

Nutritious broccoli is featured in this smooth and creamy soup with a hint of zesty lemon and a cheddar cheese upgrade.

1 1/2 lb. broccoli, cut into florets and pieces
1 medium onion, roughly chopped
3 cups low-sodium chicken or vegetable broth
Dash paprika
1 cup milk or unsweetened plain soymilk
Salt and pepper to taste

1. In a large soup pot combine the broccoli, onion, broth, paprika and Stevia drops. Bring the broccoli mixture to a boil, reduce the heat to low, and simmer until the vegetables are tender, about 25 minutes.

2. Add the milk to the soup pot and continue cooking for 2 minutes. Remove from the heat and begin ladling into a blender. Working in batches, blend until smooth and transfer to a clean saucepan.

3. Reheat the blended soup and season to taste with salt and pepper before serving.

Makes four servings, 107 calories each

Creamy Chicken Chowder

Easy to make and delectable to eat, this rich-tasting soup gets a subtle flavor boost from a surprising source.

2 strips turkey bacon, diced
1 teaspoon olive oil
1 medium onion, diced
1 medium celery stalk, diced
1 medium red bell pepper, seeded and diced
Salt to taste
1/8 teaspoon cayenne pepper, or more to taste
4 cups chicken broth
2 cups diced cooked chicken breast
1 cup unsweetened almond milk
1/8 teaspoon sugar substitute
1 teaspoon finely chopped parsley leaves

1. Fry the bacon in the oil in a heavy pot over medium heat, stirring often, until crisp. Remove bacon with a slotted spoon and drain on paper towels.

2. Add the onion, celery, bell pepper, salt, and cayenne pepper and cook over medium heat, stirring often, until vegetables are soft but not browned, about 5 minutes. Pour in the broth and bring to a boil. Reduce the heat to low and add the diced chicken. Cook on a low simmer, stirring occasionally, for 10 minutes.

3. Stir in the almond milk and sweetener and continue to cook for 3 minutes. Remove from the heat. Transfer half the soup to a blender and puree until smooth. Return to the pot and stir into the remaining soup for a creamy but still chunky consistency.

4. Taste for seasoning and serve piping hot sprinkled with the bacon bits and parsley.

Makes four servings, 272 calories each

Phase III Maintenance Recipes

Primavera Salad

Crunchy vegetables form the base of this healthy salad that's perfect for upgrading to a low carb pasta salad.

1 cup broccoli florets, cooked to crisp tender
1 cup green beans, cooked to crisp tender
1/2 medium red bell pepper, seeded and thinly sliced
1/2 cup shredded carrots
1/2 medium red onion cut into thin circles
1 cup grape tomatoes, halved
3 Tablespoons extra virgin olive oil
2 Tablespoons balsamic vinegar
1 teaspoon prepared mustard
1 small garlic clove, minced
1 Tablespoon finely chopped fresh basil leaves
1 cup diced mozzarella cheese
Salt and pepper to taste

1. In a large bowl combine the broccoli, green beans, bell pepper, carrots, red onion, and tomatoes.

2. In a small bowl whisk together olive oil, vinegar, mustard, and garlic. Pour over the vegetable mixture and toss well to coat. Stir in chopped basil, carefully fold in mozzarella, and season with salt and pepper. Serve at room temperature.

Makes four servings, 221 calories each

Chunky Guacamole

You can use this delicious and easy recipe for raw veggie dipping or as a great topping for burgers or grilled chicken.

1 ripe avocado
1 medium tomato, cored, seeded and chopped
1 small onion, finely chopped
Juice 1/2 lime
Salt and pepper to taste
Hot sauce to taste
Raw veggies for dipping

1. Cut the avocado in half and remove the seed. Using a sharp paring knife crosshatch the flesh to form small cubes. Scoop out the cubes with a spoon and transfer to a mixing bowl.

2. Add the tomato, onion, lime juice, salt, pepper, and hot sauce. Stir well to combine, mashing a bit against the sides of the bowl. Transfer to a serving dish and serve with the veggies.

Makes 4 servings, 91 calories each

Baked Goods and Desserts

Apple Crumb Pies

Apple pie is back on the menu with this simplified crustless version that's quick and delicious.

1/2 teaspoon olive oil
2 Granny Smith apples, peeled, cored, and cut into 1/4-inch thick slices
1/2 cup unsweetened applesauce
1/8 teaspoon ground cinnamon
Pinch sugar substitute
1 teaspoon lemon juice

Topping:
1/4 cup almond flour
1 Tablespoon unsalted butter, softened
1/8 teaspoon sugar substitute
Dash ground cinnamon

1. Preheat the oven to 350 degrees F. Lightly brush 2 medium-size ramekins or small pie dishes with the oil.

2. In a medium bowl combine the apples with the remaining ingredients, except those for the topping, and stir well. Spoon into each ramekin evenly. In a small bowl combine topping ingredients until the mixture resembles sand and sprinkle over each apple pie.

3. Transfer the 2 dishes to a baking sheet and bake until the apples are soft and the topping is golden, 20 to 30 minutes. Serve while still warm.

Makes two servings, 177 calories each

Grilled Peach Parfait

Use your oven broiler when grilling can't be done so as not to miss out on this delectable dessert.

2 medium peaches, halved and pitted
Dash cinnamon
1/2 cup plain nonfat yogurt
1/8 teaspoon almond extract
1/8 teaspoon sugar substitute
2 teaspoons sliced almonds

1. Heat a grill to medium-high. Slice each peach half into 4 more slices. Sprinkle all with the cinnamon.

2. Grill the peach slices until just warmed through the lightly grill marked, about 2 minutes per side. Meanwhile, combine the yogurt with the extract and sweetener.

3. To serve, alternate the grilled peaches with the yogurt in 2 parfait glasses and top each with a teaspoon of almonds.

Makes two servings, 117 calories each

Phase III Maintenance Recipes

Coconut Macaroons

Moist coconut and delicious almond flavor come together in these marvelous cookies that are perfect for any sweet craving.

1 1/3 cups unsweetened shredded coconut
1 Tablespoon almond flour
1/2 teaspoon salt
½ teaspoon almond extract
1/4 teaspoon sugar sweetener, or more to taste
2 large egg whites, beaten to foamy

1. Preheat the oven to 325 degrees F. Line a baking sheet with parchment paper.

2. In a medium bowl, toss together the coconut, almond flour and salt, distributing well. In a small bowl combine the extract with the sweetener and the egg whites. Stir the egg white mixture into the coconut mixture and drop by teaspoonfuls onto the prepared pan to form 24 cookies (close together is fine.)

3. Bake until the cookies are lightly browned on the edges, about 20 minutes. Transfer the cookies to a wire rack to cool.

Makes six servings, 59 calories each

Favorite Fruit Sorbet

Enjoy this simple recipe with a variety of seasonal fruit. If using fruit with tiny seeds, strain once pureed to remove, if desired.

2 cups diced cantaloupe, raspberries, peaches, or other fresh fruit

1 teaspoon lemon juice
1/2 teaspoon sugar substitute or more to taste
1/2 cup water

1. Place all the ingredients in a food processor and puree until smooth. Taste for the addition of more sweetener.

2. Pour into an ice cream maker and, following the manufacturer's instructions, churn until thick and creamy.

3. Transfer to an airtight container and keep frozen for up to 5 days.

Makes 4 servings, 30 calories each

Nutty Orange Scones

The delicious flavors of almonds and orange combine in these satisfying baked biscuits that are hard to resist.

1 large egg
3 Tablespoons light agave nectar
1 teaspoon orange zest
2 cups almond flour
3/4 teaspoon baking soda
Pinch of salt
1/2 cup currants
1/4 cup chopped almonds

1. Preheat the oven to 350 degrees F. Line a baking sheet with parchment paper.

2. In a medium bowl whisk together egg, agave, and orange zest. In another medium bowl whisk together almond flour, baking soda, and salt. Add egg mixture to dry mixture and stir quickly to combine. Stir in currants and almonds.

3. Drop mixture by rounded spoonfuls onto prepared baking sheet, lightly flattening and shaping with fingertips. Bake for 10 to 15 minutes or until a toothpick inserted in the center comes out clean and the tops are lightly golden.

Makes six servings, 250 calories each

Appendix: Your hCG Diet Quick Start Cookbook Bonuses

Streamline your diet with the all-on-one-page weekly menus and shopping lists—your bonuses from the *hCG Diet Quick Start Cookbook*.

Weekly menus:

Week A: Phase II VLCD — Chicken, Beef, and Seafood

Sunday

Breakfast
Coffee, tea, or water

Lunch
**Super Beef Chili
Breadstick or Melba Toast

Dinner
**Chicken with Orange and Fresh Basil
Lettuce Salad (2 cups)

Snack
Strawberries (10 medium)

Monday

Breakfast
Coffee, tea, or water

Lunch
**Chicken with Orange and Fresh Basil
Asparagus, steamed (2 cups)
Breadstick or Melba Toast

Dinner
**Tilapia with Strawberry Salsa
Spinach, steamed (3 cups raw)

Snack
Breadstick/Melba Toast

Tuesday

Breakfast
Coffee, tea, or water

Lunch
**Super Beef Chili
Breadstick or Melba Toast

Dinner
**Tilapia with Strawberry Salsa
Lettuce Salad

Snack
Apple
Breadstick/Melba Toast

Wednesday

Breakfast
Coffee, tea, or water

Lunch
**Chinese Orange Beef Stir Fry

Dinner
**Easy Chicken Cacciatore
Breadstick/Melba Toast

Snack
Strawberries (10 medium)
Breadstick/ Melba Toast

Thursday

Breakfast
Coffee, tea, or water

Lunch
**Easy Chicken Cacciatore
Breadstick/ Melba Toast

Dinner
**Chinese Orange Beef Stir Fry

Snack
1/2 Grapefruit

Friday

Breakfast
Coffee, tea, or water

Lunch
**Tangy Apple Slaw
Grilled Chicken Breast (4 oz.)

Dinner
**Broiled Lemon Garlic Shrimp
Lettuce Salad (2 cups)
Breadstick/ Melba Toast

Snack
Orange, Breadstick/ Melba Toast

Saturday

Breakfast
Coffee, tea, or water

Lunch
**Broiled Lemon Garlic Shrimp
Spinach Salad (3 cups)
Breadstick/ Melba Toast

Dinner
**The Big Bodacious Burger
**Tangy Apple Slaw

Snack
½ Grapefruit, Breadstick/ Melba Toast

The hCG Diet Quick Start Cookbook

Anne Wolfinger

www.quickstarthcg.com

Shopping lists:

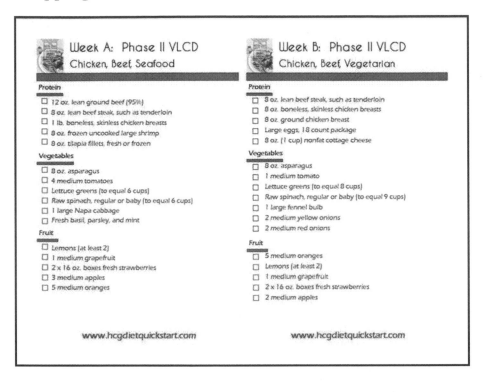

Week A: Phase II VLCD
Chicken, Beef, Seafood

Protein
- ☐ 12 oz. lean ground beef (95%)
- ☐ 8 oz. lean beef steak, such as tenderloin
- ☐ 1 lb. boneless, skinless chicken breasts
- ☐ 8 oz. frozen uncooked large shrimp
- ☐ 8 oz. tilapia fillets, fresh or frozen

Vegetables
- ☐ 8 oz. asparagus
- ☐ 4 medium tomatoes
- ☐ Lettuce greens (to equal 6 cups)
- ☐ Raw spinach, regular or baby (to equal 6 cups)
- ☐ 1 large Napa cabbage
- ☐ Fresh basil, parsley, and mint

Fruit
- ☐ Lemons (at least 2)
- ☐ 1 medium grapefruit
- ☐ 2 x 16 oz. boxes fresh strawberries
- ☐ 3 medium apples
- ☐ 5 medium oranges

www.hcgdietquickstart.com

Week B: Phase II VLCD
Chicken, Beef, Vegetarian

Protein
- ☐ 8 oz. lean beef steak, such as tenderloin
- ☐ 8 oz. boneless, skinless chicken breasts
- ☐ 8 oz. ground chicken breast
- ☐ Large eggs, 18 count package
- ☐ 8 oz. (1 cup) nonfat cottage cheese

Vegetables
- ☐ 8 oz. asparagus
- ☐ 1 medium tomato
- ☐ Lettuce greens (to equal 8 cups)
- ☐ Raw spinach, regular or baby (to equal 9 cups)
- ☐ 1 large fennel bulb
- ☐ 2 medium yellow onions
- ☐ 2 medium red onions

Fruit
- ☐ 5 medium oranges
- ☐ Lemons (at least 2)
- ☐ 1 medium grapefruit
- ☐ 2 x 16 oz. boxes fresh strawberries
- ☐ 2 medium apples

www.hcgdietquickstart.com

Download your bonuses by going to:

http://www.hcgdietquickstart.com

Happy dieting!